1992

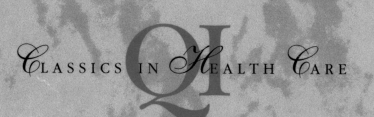
CLASSICS IN HEALTH CARE

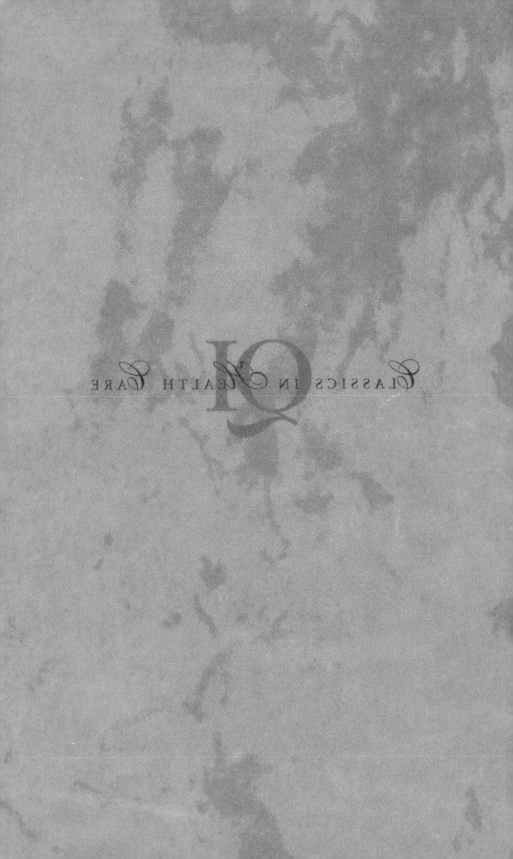

◆

STRIVING
TOWARD
IMPROVEMENT

Six Hospitals in Search of Quality

◆

Joint Commission on Accreditation of Healthcare Organizations
One Renaissance Boulevard ◆ *Oakbrook Terrace, Illinois 60181*

THE JOINT COMMISSION MISSION

The mission of the Joint Commission on Accreditation of Healthcare Organizations is to improve the quality of health care provided to the public. The Joint Commission develops standards of quality in collaboration with health professionals and others and stimulates health care organizations to meet or exceed the standards through accreditation and the teaching of quality improvement concepts.

ISBN: 0-86688-255-3
Library of Congress Number: 91-62029

Printed in the United States of America
Copyright © 1992 by the Joint Commission on Accreditation of Healthcare Organizations, Illinois

The case studies of the six hospitals profiled in this publication were written during the summer of 1991 and only reflect the hospitals' quality improvement activities up to that point.

Requests for permission to make copies of any part of this work should be mailed to Permissions Editor, Department of Publications, Joint Commission on Accreditation of Healthcare Organizations, One Renaissance Boulevard, Oakbrook Terrace, Illinois 60181.

To order copies of this publication, contact Customer Service Department, Joint Commission on Accreditation of Healthcare Organizations, One Renaissance Boulevard, Oakbrook Terrace, Illinois 60181; 708/916-5800.

Address editorial correspondence to Department of Publications, Joint Commission on Accreditation of Healthcare Organizations, One Renaissance Boulevard, Oakbrook Terrace, Illinois 60181; 708/916-5431.

Foreword

"What American managers need to learn, more than anything else," one quality expert once advised me, "is the difference between a *method* and a *result*." Obsession with results is an impediment to improvement. How could a basketball team get better if the coach taught the players, "Never take your eyes off the scoreboard?"

At first the point seems trivial—until, that is, one watches leaders do their work. Some define their roles in their organizations as battlefield commanders. "Take that hill," they say, and then manage, through accountability, control, and review, the progress toward the result. Such leaders see themselves as stewards of the end product, and they lead by reminding, exhorting, rewarding, and punishing those they lead. Their eyes are on the scoreboard.

Other leaders are different. "Forget the scoreboard for now," they say. "Study, instead, the method of play. I will teach you how to hold the ball, where to place your hands, and, better still, I will help you learn how to learn on your own." Such leaders care, of course, about results, but they are stewards of the methods through which results are won. They are not controllers; they are teachers.

When I first met Phil Ershler, I thought he was crazy. Phil is a world-class mountaineer who has stood on the summits of Everest and K2, and has climbed Aconcagua many times. He was my guide on Mount Ranier in the state of Washington—no Everest, but nonetheless a serious mountain. Rainier contains more glacier mass than any other mountain in the lower 48 states, and at its summit, 14,410 feet, the air pressure is only half that at sea level.

I had climbed to the 10,000-foot high camp on Mount Rainier three times before—a thoroughly draining, steady trudge—up 5,000 feet in just under four miles over glaring snow fields. Each time I arrived exhausted, near the limit of my sea-level lungs.

Now Phil was to guide me on a fourth climb. But first, he told us, he was going to teach us some methods. "I am going to teach you two things," he said, "how to walk and how to breathe."

We laughed. We thought we were there to learn *technique*—crampons, ice axes, crevasse rescue, not walking and breathing.

Six hours later, we were laughing no longer. Phil had done exactly what he said. The habitual, unconscious actions of walking and breathing had been transformed for us into self-conscious, planned, placed, comprehended, and practiced tools for our success on the mountain. We learned the "rest step," the use of rhythms, the conservation of motion, the focus of attention, the alternatives in placement of the foot, kicking and sliding at just the right time. We studied equipment, the shape of snow, the position of our lips and our arms, and the distances between us. Walking and breathing had become, under Phil's mentoring, not the simple, intuitive staggering and puffing of a neophyte with desperate eyes on the summit, but a constellation of a dozen or more small and purposeful parts, each designed and each defended by experience, theory, and logic. Together, these learned parts added up to a new way—a transformation of methods.

I climbed the next day to the 10,000-foot level in bright sunlight, walking and breathing a new way. I arrived tested but fresh—impossibly fresh based on my three prior experiences on the same climb. This fourth climb was different. The method had changed. Same mountain; new method. Joseph Juran would call it a "breakthrough."

Watch the six chief executive officers portrayed in this important book. If interested in quality management, you will naturally ask about the "road maps" they use—their implementation plans and their actions. But do not miss the most important point: These are leaders who have come to own the responsibility for learning, practicing, and teaching their organizations new methods to gain the summits they have always wanted.

The changes these leaders have agreed to undertake are profound; they are revising the very "walking and breathing" of management and leadership action. They are returning to basics and revising them. Michael Pugh at Parkview Episcopal Medical Center is abolishing annual merit appraisals, and John Anderson, MD, at USAF Medical Center, Wright-Patterson now regards teaching as "the natural responsibility of senior management." At Memorial Hospital and Health System, Phil Newbold is trying to encourage "unsanctioned entrepreneurship," while John Bingham at Magic Valley Regional Medical Center intends to help make his hometown the "healthiest place in America." L. Thomas Wilburn is building on a foundation of quantification and creative breakthrough he began laying at Bethesda Hospital 20 years ago. And Paul Griner, MD, and Leo Brideau are deploying Strong Memorial Hospital's research and educational capabilities to define the scope of "maximal" quality improvement.

The leaders and staff of the hospitals profiled in this book are taking the time to relearn problem solving, to study and adopt formal process improvement methods, to develop deeper understandings of and connections to present and future customers, and to reinvest in training as an organizational priority and quality as a business strategy. Each intends to make long-lasting partnerships among professionals in the health care system and to—finally—put to rest the wasteful, draining battles among physicians, administrators, nurses, and others that have too long characterized too much of medical care. Each intends to make care a true system, even if that means rethinking the very core of the hospital's social identity.

Notice the difference between *doctrine* and *discipline* in the activities of these leaders. Doctrine is absent (or at least muted), as these inventors tailor approaches to the specific histories, communities, and structures of their own organizations. But discipline is a hallmark. "By what method . . . ?" is W. Edwards Deming's recent, ringing question for those who would regain world-class quality. It doesn't take brains to aspire to the dominance of a market, the survival of a patient, or the summit of a mountain. What takes brains is the steady, scientific, *disciplined* study, learning, practice, and use of the methods through which each of those desired results is obtained.

American health care does not lack purpose. It does not lack goals, aspirations, or awareness of need. It does not need to be reminded that it exists to help or that life, comfort, dignity, and emotional peace are worth seeking. It sees the mountain that it wants to climb. Seeing it is easy.

What American health care lacks, and what most of all explains its current pain and paralysis, is confidence and mastery in a clearly defined, logically plausible, theoretically grounded, and empirically proven set of methods to attain the gains it wants. What health care lacks, and what other industries now have found, is a method for improvement. Now, in the patiently crafted and courageous examples of hospitals such as those profiled in this book, health care may once again find models that it needs to get it back, en route, upwards.

Walk and breathe. Walk and breathe. Walk and breathe. The summits are the same. Now, maybe, we can learn a way to get there.

Donald M. Berwick, MD
November 1991

Contents

An Overview of the Contents

Dozens of questions exist about implementing quality improvement (QI)* within a hospital. Many articles and books describe industry experiences with QI, and, more recently, sources have been published explaining how health care can benefit from QI and describing some successes that have been achieved.[1,2] None of these, however, provide the answers to some basic, practical implementation issues: types of structural changes an organization may need to make, resources required for staff training, the relationship between quality assurance (QA) and QI, medical staff involvement in QI, the role of leadership, and the types of behavioral changes needed in an organization. To discover how these issues are being addressed, a Joint Commission team went to the source. This team consisted of James A. Prevost, MD, Maureen P. Carr, James W. Dilley, and Maggie Kennedy. *Striving Toward Improvement* tells the stories of six hospitals making the transition to QI—the tactics they used and the barriers they ran into.

What Is QI?

QI is based on the theories of W. Edwards Deming[3,4] and Joseph Juran.[5] While working at Western Electric Laboratories in the 1930s, they discovered that variation is usually inherent in complex production processes. Deming and Juran introduced QI to post-World War II Japan, and it is credited as the method that rebuilt and revitalized the Japanese manufacturing industry. QI deemphasizes the end-of-the-

---

* *Other acronyms such as TQM (total quality management) or CQI (continuous quality improvement) are often used in the field. In this book, QI (quality improvement) will be used except when reporting the activities and ideas of the individual hospitals and their leaders. In Chapters 1-6, which describe the six hospitals, the term that each hospital prefers is used. In Chapter 8, which transcribes the roundtable discussion among the hospital leaders, the terms are used according to each participant's preference.*

line "inspection" approach common to most organizations and concentrates instead on the description, measurement, and constant improvement of key processes. It assumes that systems and processes, not people, are at the root of most quality problems. QI is a proactive approach that minimizes the potential for future errors rather than focusing on the resolution of problems after they have occurred—quality is designed into products and services. Organizations committed to QI continuously improve performance to better meet customer needs.

Faced with growing foreign competition over the past decade, American industry has become concerned with meeting customer needs, the complexity of production processes and variation within them, the failure of inspection to improve quality, and the cost of poor quality. Quality improvement has been reimported as a method to attack such problems. The Malcolm Baldrige National Quality Award, established in 1987, is the prime example of this national initiative to improve the quality of American products and services. It describes the basic principles of QI and, through a rigorous assessment process, finds and recognizes companies that excel in quality management.

While a hospital and a manufacturing plant appear to have little in common, experts in industrial quality control who serve as consultants to hospitals report "that health care is just as riddled with operational defects as any other industry they have studied."[6] Both the clinical care provided directly to patients and all the governance, management, and support processes that surround these are amenable to the method of QI. The health care field and industry share another trait—both are operated by people. Many of the theories behind QI are behavioral and address ways in which people perform best within an organization.

Since Deming's and Juran's initial efforts, a number of other experts have contributed their theories of QI, including Philip Crosby,[7] AV Feigenbaum,[8] and Kaoru Ishikawa.[9] While the experts may differ in their approaches to QI, a number of common characteristics are shared by all:

- QI is driven by the leaders of the organization. Active involvement of all leaders, including the chief executive officer, board members, and senior management, is essential. In health care, physicians, nurses, and other clinical leaders should be involved. These leaders create an environment that focuses on quality, frees staff to improve and assess processes across departments and disciplines, and encourages change and new ideas.

2

- Customer-supplier relationships are developed and understood. QI organizations attempt to understand the needs of their customers and design processes that will consistently meet or exceed those needs. Organizations see themselves as part of a larger customer-supplier chain. Suppliers provide inputs to a process, which in turn delivers outputs to customers. These concepts are applied to both the organization's external and internal relationships. Initially, thinking of patients and fellow staff members as customers can be a language barrier in health care, but acceptance of this concept can lead to the successful exploration of important processes that affect patient care.

- A move away from inspection-based management to the improvement of processes is occurring. QI concentrates on variations in important processes and attempts to identify and control the source of variation. For example, in health care organizations, staff would focus on key processes that affect patient care, including direct clinical care and governance, management, and support services. Defects in these processes result in waste, rework, and increased costs. Referred to as the 85/15 theory, Deming concludes that 85% of the problems detected within an organization are process related or system related (a system being a group of related processes). Only 15% can be traced to the individual worker. This contrasts with many peer review and QA approaches used in health care today.

- All employees are involved in the exploration of processes. QI recognizes that many individuals within an organization contribute to positive outcomes. Frequently, cross-discipline or cross-departmental teams are formed to explore processes and each person contributes specific knowledge about his or her aspect of the process.

- Formal problem-solving methods and statistical tools are used. Most organizations adopt a problem-solving method to guide process improvement efforts. While methods vary, most are based on the Shewhart cycle illustrated in Figure 1 (page 4). Various components of a process are measured in QI, including customer needs, inputs and outputs, and the characteristics of the process. There is a reliance on data for decision-making, and a number of QI tools are used to collect and analyze data. These include flowcharts, cause-and-effect diagrams, Pareto charts, and control charts. Appendix A (page 255) provides an overview of QI tools.

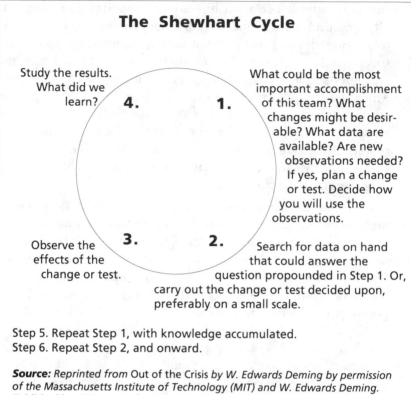

The various problem-solving methods that the hospitals in this book use are all based on the Shewhart Cycle.

The text within the figure reads:

The Shewhart Cycle

Study the results. What did we learn? **4.**

1. What could be the most important accomplishment of this team? What changes might be desirable? What data are available? Are new observations needed? If yes, plan a change or test. Decide how you will use the observations.

Observe the effects of the change or test. **3.**

2. Search for data on hand that could answer the question propounded in Step 1. Or, carry out the change or test decided upon, preferably on a small scale.

Step 5. Repeat Step 1, with knowledge accumulated.
Step 6. Repeat Step 2, and onward.

Source: Reprinted from Out of the Crisis by W. Edwards Deming by permission of the Massachusetts Institute of Technology (MIT) and W. Edwards Deming. Published by MIT, Center for Advanced Engineering Study, Cambridge, MA 02138. © 1988 by W. Edwards Deming.

Figure 1. The various problem-solving methods that the hospitals in this book use are all based on the Shewhart Cycle.

The Development of the Book

Selection of the six hospitals profiled in this book began in January 1991. Through networking, 60 hospitals currently engaged in QI were initially identified. It was a diverse sample with a range in hospital type and size. The 60 hospitals were grouped by the following stratification:

- Community hospitals with an average census of
  —less than 100 beds,
  —100–250 beds,
  —250–500 beds, and
  —500–1,000 beds;
- Military hospitals; and

4

• Academic health centers.

This stratified list was then separately reviewed by four national QI experts: Donald Berwick, MD, of the National Demonstration Project in Brookline, Massachusetts; Paul Batalden, MD, of the Hospital Corporation of America in Nashville, Tennessee; and Kathryn Johnson and Hannah King of the Healthcare Forum in San Francisco. They were asked to identify the hospitals in each of the six categories that were the most actively involved in QI. Based on this information, the list was narrowed to 20 hospitals.

The 20 hospitals were then contacted about the project. Nineteen of the 20 agreed to participate in the next step of the selection process—a structured telephone interview. A questionnaire (see Appendix B, page 267) was constructed that would help obtain information regarding the extent of each hospital's QI activities, including the degree of hospitalwide QI involvement, leadership role in QI, strategic quality planning, problem-solving processes used, QI training provided to staff, human resource utilization, and quality results. This questionnaire was formulated based on the knowledge obtained from organizational change research and literature reviews on QI. Each interview lasted approximately one hour and involved the chief executive officer of each hospital and/or other key staff.

From the information obtained during this interview, the 19 hospitals were evaluated. To provide the reader with information on a range of topics related to QI, the team needed to identify those hospitals whose QI efforts were fairly advanced. Another important aspect of the selection process was to identify each hospital's unique features or approaches that would provide varying perspectives on QI to the reader (for example, a unique vision or strategy, a different problem-solving method). There was no attempt to identify the "best" QI hospitals; rather, the objective was to identify hospitals that were well along in their transition and showed a diversity of transition strategies. With this in mind, the following criteria were devised to evaluate each hospital's inclusion in the book:

• Length of time involved in QI;

• Degree of staff training;

• Use of teams;

• Governing body involvement;

• Integration of QA and QI;

• Use of QI methods and tools;

- QI supports (for example, information systems, personnel system);
- Measurable results;
- Application to clinical process;
- Physician involvement;
- Application of principles and methods with vendors and payers;
- "Benchmarking"; and
- Unique aspects and features.

Based on these criteria, the six hospitals profiled in this book were selected for on-site visits.

What This Book Will Provide

During the two days spent at each hospital, the application of QI principles was observed first-hand, leaders and staff were interviewed, team meetings were observed, and the questions asked during the telephone interview were explored in greater depth. Hospital staff described the barriers they had encountered during their transition to QI and the lessons they had learned. They described how their jobs had changed and shared the successes they had achieved using QI methods.

Chapters 1–6 provide case studies of each hospital's journey toward QI. While each chapter tries to capture the unique culture and flavor of each hospital, all six chapters follow the same outline format:

- *Description and Demographics.* This section describes the hospital's patient population, number of beds, ownership, and other pertinent demographic information.

- *History.* The steps the hospital took in implementing QI are described in this section.

- *Philosophy.* This section describes the QI theories and concepts to which the hospital subscribes.

- *Strategy.* This section explains the hospital's methods and plans for implementing QI, including the long-range objectives and/or issues on which the hospital focuses.

- *QI Process.* The problem-solving approach that the hospital has adopted is explained in this section, as well as the hospital's method for chartering teams, examples of QI team activities, and a case study of a QI team's efforts.

- *QA/QI Relationship.* The approach that the hospital is taking toward integrating QA and QI is discussed.

- *Education.* The hospital's methods for training staff in QI concepts and tools are explained in this section.

- *QI Supports.* QI hospitals need to address several theoretical and practical issues, such as attaining customer feedback, providing process-related data to staff, and rewarding team efforts. The hospital's progress in these areas is addressed in "QI Supports"; other issues may also be addressed when applicable to a particular hospital.

- *Physician Involvement.* The hospital's approach to enlisting physician support in QI activities is covered in this section.

This outline format will allow readers to compare and contrast the techniques and strategies each hospital is using to implement QI and to quickly identify specific information needed.

After visiting the hospitals, it became apparent that they shared many of the same experiences and ran into many of the same barriers. While the first six chapters focus on what is unique about each hospital, Chapter 7 concentrates on the common experiences of all the hospitals profiled.

After the site visits, the leaders of each hospital were brought together for a roundtable discussion of the issues that came up during the visits, including the changes that occur in leadership roles within a QI organization, the general sequence of transitional steps for achieving QI in hospitals, and aspects of QI that interest physicians. Chapter 8 is a transcript of that discussion. It expands on the material in Chapters 1–6.

Chapter 9 looks toward the future of QI and identifies those issues that may have a potential impact on hospitals implementing QI in the future.

An epilogue has been added to the book to address a concern of many hospitals—continuing to meet Joint Commission requirements while undertaking the immense task of moving an organization toward QI.

What is *not* provided in this book is the "best" method for implementing QI or the "right" approaches to such issues as integrating QA and QI or approaching the medical staff with QI. It is not possible to tell what is right for a particular organization. Instead, this book tries to provide an understanding of the general steps hospitals go through when implementing QI. The experiences and barriers recounted on these pages should help other health care organizations identify potential strategies for implementing QI and avoid some of the difficulties others have encountered.

Conclusion

The six hospitals profiled in this publication represent the many hospitals across the country that are "striving toward improvement" in these times of fiscal constraints and increased demands for quality. Armed with the concepts and tools of QI, these hospitals are attempting to meet the challenges facing health care in the coming years. A wonderful characteristic of those involved in QI is their propensity to share information. This book would not have been possible without the assistance and kindness of the leaders and staff in the six hospitals. They were all excellent and patient teachers and very generously shared the mistakes they made during their transition as well as their successes. The lessons and strategies shared in this book should help other organizations in their strides toward quality.

References

1. Berwick D, Godfrey AB, Roessner J: *Curing Health Care.* San Francisco: Jossey-Bass, 1990.
2. Berwick D: Continuous improvement as the ideal in health care. *N Engl J Med* 320: 53–56, 1989.
3. Deming WE: *Out of the Crisis.* Cambridge, MA: Massachusetts Institute of Technology Press, 1986.
4. Walton M: *The Deming Management Method.* New York: Putnam Publishing Group, 1986.
5. Juran JM: *Quality Control Handbook.* New York: McGraw-Hill, 1988.
6. Berwick DM: Health services research and quality of care. Assignments for the 1990s. *Med Care* 27(8): 763–771, 1989.
7. Crosby PM: *Quality Is Free.* New York: McGraw-Hill, 1979.
8. Feigenbaum AV: *Total Quality Control.* New York: McGraw-Hill, 1983.
9. Ishikawa K: *What is Total Quality Control?* Englewood Cliffs, NJ: Prentice-Hall, 1985.

1 Panning for Quality
Parkview Episcopal Medical Center
Pueblo, Colorado

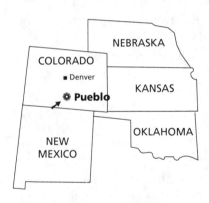

Type of hospital: Not-for-profit community
Scope of services: General medical/surgical
Beds: 305, with average census of 135
Extent of QI involvement: Having begun their QI activities in 1988, the chief executive officer describes Parkview as being on "the bleeding edge, which is what happens to hospitals on the cutting edge." One hundred percent of hospital departments are using QI techniques in some form, and teams are investigating processes throughout the hospital for improvement, including five hospitalwide systems identified by leaders

Special aspects of Parkview's QI activities:
— A culture change has taken place—quality has become part of daily work
— Data and QI structure have empowered staff
— The traditional merit system has been eliminated
— Staff share a restlessness with the status quo
— Measures have been established to determine the success of the hospital's objectives
— QI efforts are focused along five hospitalwide systems

More than 100 years after the last gold was stripped from the Colorado mines, Michael Pugh uncovered Pueblo's richest strain— the spirit those gold diggers left behind. When Pugh arrived as president and chief executive officer of Parkview Episcopal Medical Center, the community was facing economic challenges similar to many industry-driven communities in the 1980s; 4,800 people had been laid off by CF&I Steel, the town's largest employer. Once the

"Pittsburgh of the West," Pueblo was crippled. But the town "picked itself up by the bootstraps," according to Abel Chavez, chairman of Parkview's board. New businesses have been recruited, and the economy is beginning to turn around. "The whole community took on a new attitude toward making change happen," Chavez says. This same attitude pervaded Parkview. Economic survival made change a necessity for the hospital—95% of Parkview's patients are either Medicare or Medicaid, members of health maintenance or preferred provider organizations, or medically indigent. Pugh saw quality improvement (QI) as the means to make change happen, and in 1988 the hospital embarked on a commitment to QI. Three years later a cultural change has begun to occur at Parkview; QI is not a program here but is embedded in staff's daily activities. It is QI's leader-driven structure that facilitated a cultural change. When Pugh handed his staff a process-improvement approach, trained them in QI methods and tools, expected them to argue with data not opinion, and set up a Quality Forum for sharing ideas and opportunities, he provided a structure that essentially empowered staff to creatively approach problems and opportunities for improvement.

Staff at Parkview cannot wait to talk about the discoveries they have made flowcharting a process or describe the barriers they have broken by treating other disciplines as customers. There are so many storyboards around the hospital they appear to be holding up the walls. Nothing excites staff members more than describing a process they have been doing wrong for years. Speak to Mike Del Priore, director of cardiopulmonary services, and he glows about the drastic reduction in unacceptable sputum tests (from 12% to 5%), or stop by Rosalie Glenn's office, director of food service, and she will pull out her control charts that show the reduction in undelivered food trays to patients. The top-to-bottom integration of QI is emphasized by Parkview's Quality Forum, a meeting held every two weeks at which teams present their stories to the QI Council (QIC). One nursing director, Paula Grassmick, speaks of key quality characteristics, theories of variation, and customer needs when presenting the story of her intravenous feeding team as though speaking in her original tongue. There is a spirit of entrepeneurship, of freedom at Parkview. According to CW Smith, chief operating officer, "QI provides a means to cause change as opposed to waiting for change to happen. QI is a way to self-determination."

Description and Demographics

The architecture of the storefronts reveals Pueblo's history as a frontier town. Situated about 110 miles from Denver, at the confluence of Fountain Creek and the Arkansas River, this region became a natural crossroads for Spanish conquistadors, Indians, mountain men, traders, and trappers. In the 1840s, fur traders built Fort Pueblo, which was later abandoned after an Indian massacre in 1854. Four years later gold brought settlers scurrying over the mountains, and Pueblo was officially born. Today over 100,000 people live in Pueblo. Since the steel mill laid off a large percentage of the population, Pueblo is slowly making the transition from being a blue collar community to a service community. Major employers include Unisys, McDonnell-Douglas Astronautics, and CF&I. Pueblo's weather attracts significant tourist business as well (winter temperatures stay above 50° F, and the sun shines 76% of the time).

One of two community hospitals in Pueblo, Parkview is a 305-bed, not-for-profit hospital with an average census of 135. Primarily an acute medical/surgical hospital, Parkview also has a large behavioral medicine program. Parkview has captured a large percentage of the Medicaid psychiatric business due to demographics and an overspill of patients from nearby Colorado State Hospital. Eighty percent of Parkview's adult chronically ill and 50% of all behavioral medicine patients are on Medicaid. The medical staff consists of more than 210 physicians. Major services include behavioral medicine, computerized tomography scan lab, cardiology, chemical dependency, emergency, pharmacy, neurological care, laboratory, and rehabilitation services. Parkview's outpatient services, which include medical/surgical, same-day surgery, emergency, and home care, have been steadily growing as well.

The hospital board has a management contract with Quorum Health Resources, formerly known as Hospital Corporation of America (HCA) Management Company. Quorum, a hospital management company located in Nashville, Tennessee, is enthusiastically encouraging the hospitals it manages to make the transition to QI. Parkview is a role model for Quorum hosptials. As a result, Parkview is able to take advantage of many consulting, educational, and networking opportunities that Quorum provides.

History

Pugh was introduced to the concepts of W. Edwards Deming at a crucial point in his career. In 1988, he had been a hospital administrator for ten years and had reached a turning point. While he had been successful to that point, Pugh was tired of continually fighting fires. He was asked by HCA to attend an introductory class on QI taught by Paul Batalden, MD, in April 1988. The theories of Deming he learned that day "captured his imagination." He went home to Pueblo committed to changing Parkview to a QI-based organization. Always a risk-taker, Pugh was certain at first that he would be able to change the culture at Parkview in 18 months, less than half the time predicted by experts.

Pugh admits to "treading water a lot" in the beginning. Operating at first under the critical mass theory (that is, "keep educating people and something will happen"), Pugh immediately began educating senior and middle management and the board on the concepts of QI. Soon after staff were encouraged to form teams. These initial team efforts met with mixed success. Many of the processes chosen for investigation were too complex; some were actually systems of processes. For example, Pugh described a medication floor stock team that developed "a cause-and-effect diagram the size of a wall, but didn't get anywhere." Teams also lacked sufficient education in QI methods and team dynamics. An early team looking into the audiovisual process believed a democratic process was all that was needed for success. Essentially, "the team fought for eight or nine months," according to Pugh, and concluded they needed $4,000 in additional audiovisual equipment.

From these early struggles, Pugh and his staff learned that educating a critical mass was not enough and that staff needed more direction and focus. During 1989 and 1990, senior management concentrated on focusing and developing a structure for Parkview's QI initiatives. Once a focus and direction was provided, Parkview's QI activities began taking off at a rapid speed. The following are some of the significant accomplishments during this two-year period:

- *Drafting Parkview's quality statements.* After a four-month strategic planning process, Parkview's senior management and board adopted a five-year vision and strategic plan. Part of this process was translating Deming's 14 points to reflect the hospital's own philosophy (see Table 1.1, page 13). Staff consider this a key step in developing the philosophical framework for Parkview's organizational transformation.

Table 1.1. Parkview's Quality Statements

1. Parkview's mission statement will continue to govern our direction in pursuing the continuous improvement of all services. This commitment to quality and service is the most important of our guidelines.

2. Parkview management will study and learn the philosophy of continuous improvement and lead the transformation.

3. We will continue to meet external inspection requirements such as the Joint Commission, Health Department, state, Medicare, Medicaid and others. However, we believe that building quality into the design of systems is better than inspection.

4. Value is determined by price and quality. We seek suppliers who will be our long-term partners and who will provide us the best service and products at the lowest total cost.

5. We seek to define and continuously improve every process of planning, operations, and service delivery.

6. We believe all employees must have a clear understanding of their jobs and their role in the organization.

7. We are committed to leadership that focuses on the improvement of the systems in which people work.

8. We are committed to the development of an organizational environment that is free of fear and that is characterized by trust and integrity.

9. We are committed to the elimination of barriers that impair teamwork and create waste, rework, and needless complexity.

10. We believe people want to do a good job and are motivated in an environment where suggestions are acted upon, ideas are shared, and teamwork flourishes.

11. We believe in creating budgets and numeric estimates to guide and assess our progress based on the capacity of the organization to achieve its goals.

12. It is the responsibility of leadership to create an organizational culture that allows pride of workmanship. Employees must be given the necessary resources to produce quality work.

13. We believe our employees are our greatest asset. We support and encourage our employees in their efforts to seek personal and professional development.

14. Success in the quality improvement process depends on the involvement, cooperation, and enthusiasm of every board member, employee, physician, supplier, patient, and customer.

Source: *Reprinted with permission from Parkview Episcopal Medical Center, Pueblo, Colorado, 1991.*

- *Merging QIC meetings with executive staff meetings.* Originally Pugh and the rest of senior management met separately as a QIC to discuss QI initiatives and as a senior management team to decide operational issues. In what Pugh and his staff consider a major paradigm shift, the two meetings were merged into the QIC meeting about midway through 1989. The merging of the two meetings emphasized that quality is a part of day-to-day activities. Now all the operations of the organization are dealt with "in the context of quality," Pugh says. For example, the hospital is undergoing the second phase of a major construction project. By approaching it from a quality perspective, planning with the people who will work in the new area is more emphasized than it would have been before QI.

- *Attaining greater technical and educational assistance.* An important position on the QIC was created in 1989—a full-time QI coach, BJ Ivey, reports directly to Pugh and is responsible for developing QI training programs for staff. At about the same time, a statistical consultant was employed to provide training in statistical process control, and a QI fellow from Quorum joined Parkview staff for nine months.

- *Reorganizing the management structure.* Parkview created two patient service divisions and merged the nursing departments and the ancillary and support departments together within the same divisions. Each division is headed by a vice-president of patient services who reports directly to the chief operating officer. Both vice-presidents are registered nurses. This new structure has been instrumental in breaking down traditional barriers between nursing and other departments and has allowed departments to more clearly understand their customer/supplier role.

- *Developing the second phase of its "rollout" plan.* To guide its QI activities, Parkview developed an implementation or "rollout" plan. This plan has had two phases to date. The initial plan concentrated primarily on education of staff in QI concepts. Phase II of Parkview's rollout plan is more specific. It identifies specific tasks that staff at different levels of the organization (for example, board, QIC, departments) should accomplish and defines five hospitalwide systems (for example, admission, food service) where staff are concentrating their QI efforts (see "Strategy").

When Pugh introduced QI to Parkview, the prevailing thought among department managers was "this too shall pass." The test of whether QI was a fad or a true commitment came in late 1989 when the hospital ran into extreme financial difficulties caused by Medicare/Medicaid cutbacks, poor performance of HMO contracts, and an unusual number of medically indigent and Medicare outliers. Parkview lost $1 million from November to December in 1989. According to Pugh, "It essentially came down to a decision that money had to be saved *now.*" Department managers "thought this was it, the end of the QI," Eileen Dennis, vice-president, patient services, says. But no jobs were lost and the commitment of senior management to QI remained. Senior management used QI concepts and tools to find the areas of waste and immediate savings.

As they approach the four-year anniversary of their QI efforts, Pugh has become much more conservative: "At least four years to life," he says now, predicting how long it takes to achieve a cultural transformation. And he doesn't promise he won't "change that to five years to life" by next year.

Philosophy

Pugh believes one has to look at the "big picture" to make lasting changes with QI. As illustrated in Figure 1.1 (page 15) Pugh considers three characteristics necessary to QI: organizational/cultural transformation, process knowledge, and customer knowledge. This "big picture" is closely linked to Deming's chain reaction (which concludes that quality costs less):

Improve quality → Costs decrease → Productivity improves →

Capture market → Stay in business → Provide more jobs

Once an organization makes a commitment to quality and begins listening to customer needs and improving the processes that are important to those customers, Deming theorizes that customer satisfaction and productivity/profitability will go up.

Pugh sees the Deming model as a method to fight hospital costs. Pugh has a "gut fact" (which is what he calls a gut feeling one has for more than two years) that 25%–50% of all hospital costs are the result of systems that create waste, rework, needless complexity, malpractice medicine, and wrong clinical decisions (malpractice medicine and wrong clinical decisions being the lowest portion of this percentage). Pugh cites billing and data processing clerks as examples since they are continually straightening out mistakes. He believes the percentage of rework is probably higher in health care than in other industries,

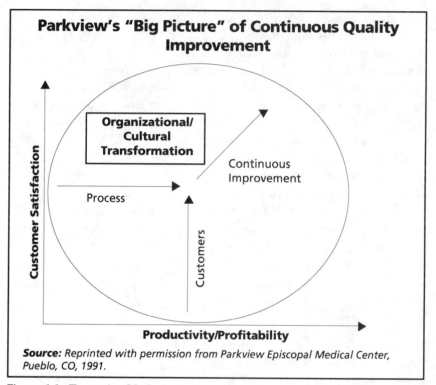

Figure 1.1. To attain QI, Parkview is combining customer knowledge, process knowledge, and organizational transformation. As a result, staff expect profits, productivity, and customer satisfaction to increase.

estimating it to be 20%–30%, since hospital systems have evolved rather than having been planned. Pugh believes that the solution to rising health care costs rests with the hospitals, that hospitals need to improve their processes and systems to reduce costs rather than "looking for someone to bail us out." Pugh believes that hospitals have always accepted waste, rework, and needless complexity as the way things work. "If we could [eliminate] 5% of the costs of rework, we'd be in a better position," he says. Pugh sees QI, with its emphasis on process improvement, as the means to reduce rework.

This point of view has made Pugh unpopular with some in health care. Staff recognize that the reduction of rework and the improvement of processes might translate into lost jobs, particularly at the middle management and line level. Although Deming's chain reaction promises the creation of new jobs, existing jobs will undoubtedly be eliminated by streamlining processes. Pugh stresses Parkview's commitment to locating new jobs for those who are displaced as a result of QI efforts. If staff "think their jobs will be eliminated and they would be on the street, then the QI effort is gone," Pugh says.

Another part of the QI philosophy at Parkview is the link Pugh sees between clinical and operational functions. Senior management decided up-front to wait to use QI tools and methods in clinical areas of the hospital. This decision was driven, in part, by the belief that operational functions directly affect clinical functions. Pugh believes that reducing the variation in operational processes will reduce the variation in clinical processes. For example, it is difficult for a cardiac catheterization to be successful unless such processes as admission, scheduling, diagnostic x-ray, transport, and lab and diagnostic cardiology are performed accurately and on a timely basis. Variation in these processes can and will affect the outcome of the cardiac catheterization. "Clinical won't work properly unless operational is working," Pugh says. Parkview decided to make "the leap of faith that physicians know what they're doing," Pugh says, and work on those operational processes that affect clinical areas first. Figure 1.2 (below) illustrates this view. As explained further in "Physician Involvement,"

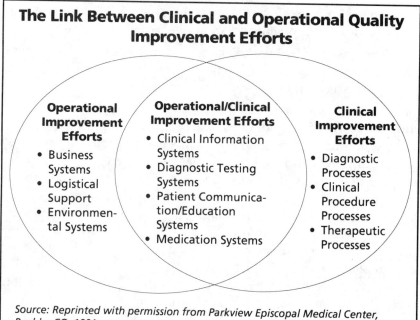

The Link Between Clinical and Operational Quality Improvement Efforts

Operational Improvement Efforts
- Business Systems
- Logistical Support
- Environmental Systems

Operational/Clinical Improvement Efforts
- Clinical Information Systems
- Diagnostic Testing Systems
- Patient Communication/Education Systems
- Medication Systems

Clinical Improvement Efforts
- Diagnostic Processes
- Clinical Procedure Processes
- Therapeutic Processes

Source: Reprinted with permission from Parkview Episcopal Medical Center, Pueblo, CO, 1991.

Figure 1.2. Because of the link between clinical and operational systems, staff at Parkview believe the hospital's clinical systems will improve as a result of their QI efforts on the operational side of the hospital.

other reasons for postponing the involvement of physicians included not wanting clinicians to confuse QI with QA and wanting to gain credibility with physicians by improving systems that affected their daily work life.

Strategy

Parkview's organizationwide strategic plan is linked directly to the vision of becoming "the regional leader in providing and developing quality health care services that exceed the expectations of our customers." Senior management and the board identified four important objectives that would help them reach this vision:

- *Customers.* Be the health care system of choice for patients, medical staff and allied health professionals, third-party payers, and health care employees.

- *Financial performance.* Have the financial strength to weather external economic and industry pressures, maintain Parkview's commitment to QI, and continuously improve our systems, processes, facilities, technology, and organizational culture.

- *Quality improvement.* Parkview's QI philosophy and methods are supported and practiced systemwide as part of daily work life.

- *Innovation and leadership.* Parkview is an innovator and leader and will be recognized for QI, development of health care programs and services, and community participation.

Each year, senior management develop a management plan that includes specific tasks staff need to accomplish under each objective.

To support their strategy, Parkview needed a plan to guide their QI effort. Parkview's initial QI rollout plan, developed at the start of the hospital's QI efforts, primarily concentrated on hospitalwide education and awareness. As discussed earlier, it soon became apparent that education alone could not create a QI organization; staff needed focus and direction. With the help of Phyllis Virgil, a QI fellow from Quorum who spent nine months at Parkview, staff developed Phase II of their rollout plan in January 1990. Important to the implementation of the rollout plan was the involvement of senior leadership in its development. All QIC members participated in developing the contents of the rollout plan in some capacity. This participatory process allowed the QIC to have a strong sense of ownership and enthusiasm for the plan.

Staff expectations. The rollout plan identifies education-related tasks that individuals at different levels of the organization (for example,

QIC, board, medical staff, department managers, and staff) are expected to accomplish. As shown in Figure 1.3 (pages 20 –21) each task is coded according to level of expectation ("must do," "should do," "nice to do") and difficulty ("basic," "intermediate," "advanced"). For example, QIC members must use cause-and-effect diagrams, Pareto charts, checklists, run charts, and other QI tools; board members should participate in role model hospital visits; and departments must identify their key customers and begin to investigate a process that is important to those customers.

Rollout of QI in this manner encourages the "practice of QI theory and tools in the daily work life of all employees." For example, as part of their department activities, pharmacy staff asked the nurses— whom they identified as one of their key customers—how pharmacy could help them. The nurses pointed out a major problem with medication carts they were receiving from pharmacy. Medication carts, which hold each patient's daily medications, were routinely filled by the pharmacy 24 hours before being sent to the patient floor. During those 24 hours, changes in patient medication frequently occurred. Although pharmacy routinely ran catch-up lists to update the medication carts before delivery, cart-filling errors continued. However, the pharmacy did not know the seriousness of the problem until they asked the nurses. "Pharmacy didn't know that nursing always fixed the problem before," Pugh says. The pharmacy began tracking its data to understand the process and suggested changing the cart fill time to just five hours prior to delivery and eliminating all catch-up lists but one. As a result, the pharmacy charted an eightfold decrease in cart-filling errors. No formal team effort was involved in this instance; management recognized a problem by talking to the customer and tracked the cause through data. The paradigm shift that occurred when staff recognized their fellow staff as customers led to improvements in the exchanges between departments and individuals.

Strategic focus. Also identified in the rollout plan are the specific areas where the hospital is focusing its QI efforts. Based on customer feedback, five systems were designated:

- Admissions;
- Charging;
- Billing;
- Dietary; and

A Cross-Section from Parkview's Roll-Out Plan
Quality Improvement Council Practice

Code	Must Do	Responsibility	Time
MB*	Use meeting skills	CEO	Each QIC meeting
MB	Preplan meeting process —use during meetings	CEO/QIC members as responsible for agenda item	Each QIC meeting
MB	Flowchart processes	CEO/QIC	Ongoing
MB	Use cause-and-effect diagrams	CEO/QIC	Ongoing
MB	Use Pareto charts	CEO/QIC	Ongoing
MB	Use checklists	CEO/QIC	Ongoing
MB	Use histograms	CEO/QIC	Ongoing
MB	Use run chart and control chart	CEO/QIC	Ongoing
MB	Use sound data collection methods to plot data over time	CEO/QIC	Ongoing
MB	Provide feedback to coach	CEO/QIC	Ongoing

• *The first letter in the code stands for the level of expectation (for example, "M" means "must do"). The second letter represents the difficulty of the task (for example, "B" means "basic" and "I" means "intermediate").*

• Clinical results reporting.

Management made it clear that every department in the hospital connected to these systems should be involved in the improvement process. As explained in "QI Process," systems teams have been formed to begin investigating these five areas. Systems are sets of interrelated processes. While staff are also encouraged to identify and improve processes outside the five focus areas, either through teams or using problem solving in daily activities, priority is given to these areas.

Recently two additional systems of focus were identified for hospitalwide QI efforts: the environmental system, which involves improving all the processes that contribute to the facility appearance (housekeeping, maintenance, construction), and the patient care delivery system, which involves defining the best current method of

A Cross-Section from Parkview's
Roll-Out Plan (continued)

Code	Must Do	Responsibility	Time
MB	Use leadership skills: model the way, share inspired vision, encourage the heart, challenge the process, enable others to act	CEO/QIC	Ongoing
MB	Share successes/ celebrate	CEO/QIC	Ongoing
MB	Give book/article/ chapter reports at QIC meetings	CEO/QIC	One per year QIC members
MI	Use FOCUS-PDCA on actual process 1. One QIC process 2. Individual process	CEO/QIC	By 4th quarter

Source: *Reprinted with permission from Parkview Episcopal Medical Center, Pueblo, CO, 1991.*

Figure 1.3. In Parkview's rollout plan, staff are assigned tasks they "must do," "should do," and those that would be "nice to do." The figure above provides a cross-section from the tasks the QIC "must" accomplish.

delivering clinical care to patients. Initially, Parkview is looking at cardiology patients and pneumonia patients with this system approach.

Recognizing the importance of gauging the success of their QI initiatives, Parkview developed several measurement tools, which are linked to their vision for the future. As part of an exercise, senior management identified the key quality characteristics of the "future" Parkview. Once these characteristics were decided on, management determined measurement tools and measurement frequency. Table 1.2 (page 22) lists Parkview's quality measurements.

QI Process

Team activities are either connected to the five focus areas, which the QIC has identified as priority efforts (see "Strategy"), or are formed by

21

Table 1.2. Parkview's Hospitalwide Key Quality Characteristics

Key Quality Characteristic	Measurement Tool	Measurement Frequency
1. Which is the best hospital? (Physician)	Physician Hospital Quality Trend Survey	Annually
2. Which is the best hospital? (Community)	SRI/Gallup	Two years
3. Overall quality care (Physician)	Physician Hospital Quality Trend Survey	Annually
4. Overall quality care (Patient)	Patient Hospital Quality Trend Survey	Biannually
5. Would return (Patient)	Patient Hospital Quality Trend Survey	Biannually
6. Overall satisfaction (Employee)	Employee Hospital Quality Trend Survey	Annually
7. Net days accounts receivable	Financial Reports	Monthly
8. Income from operations	Financial Reports	Monthly
9. Cost per adjusted admission	Financial Reports	Monthly
10. Employee turnover rate	Financial Reports	Monthly

Source: *Reprinted with permission from Parkview Episcopal Medical Center, Pueblo, Colorado, 1991*

staff interested in investigating a process that is close to them. Informal teams are numerous and successful, such as the first-case operating room QI team, which reduced the delay of morning surgery start from 180 minutes a week to 45 minutes a week. Initially, staff had to go through the QIC to charter a team, but the QIC did away with this process because it was too burdensome and members were afraid it would discourage staff from taking the initiative in improvement efforts.

For each of the five systems, a core team coordinates the intradepartmental and interdepartmental QI efforts within that focus area. Due to the complexity of each system, many teams operate within one focus area to investigate the many processes that comprise that system. For example, the clinical results reporting team began by investigating the reporting of electroencephalogram (EEG) results, which is just one interdepartmental process in the clinical results reporting system. Feeding into the EEG process are many department-specific processes that also need investigating, such as in the lab and radiology. Intradepartmental teams were set up within these departments to improve these specific processes as well; these intradepartmental teams report back to the main QI team. This structure forces departments to identify relationships with their internal customers and understand how processes involve many disciplines. A case study (below) provides a more complete explanation of the work the admissions system team has completed.

An important structural element that helps these system teams work is that each system is "championed" by a member of the QIC. This structure ensures that each system improvement effort is owned and coached by a member of senior leadership. So not only did senior managers contribute to the rollout plan, they also helped guide its implementation. The champions lead the main system teams, work with department managers and employees in problem solving, secure

(continued on page 32)

Case Study
A Systems Approach: Applying QI Tools and Methods to Improve a Hospital's Admission System

The following case study shares the experiences of the Parkview team that was established to improve our admissions system. Systems improvement requires "systems-thinking"—a discipline for seeing dynamic interrelationships rather than fragmented parts, for seeing processes of change rather than snapshots in time. Peter Senge describes systems thinking as "a conceptual framework, a body of knowledge and tools that has been developed over the past fifty years, to make the full patterns clearer, and to help us see how to change them effectively...."[1] We applied QI thinking, tools, and methods to clarify and understand the interrelated processes in our admissions system and select strategies for improvement. The FOCUS-PDCA framework, demonstrated on pages 34–35, will be used to tell our story.

Find a system to improve. Based on feedback from patients, employees, physicians, and payers, Parkview's Quality Improvement Council chose the admissions system as one system of organizational focus.

Organize a team that knows the system. A core team was established to guide system clarification, understanding, and selection of improvement strategies. Core team members include

- Donna Wheeler, Director of Admissions;
- Katrina Van Hoesen, Vice-President Strategic Planning and Marketing;
- BJ Ivey, Quality Improvement Coach; and
- Marcus Padgett, QI Consultant.

At later stages, the core team brought in others as consultants, including other departments and physicians' offices.

The core team developed an opportunity statement to clarify the admission system and its boundaries and to identify why improvement was needed. This opportunity statement is provided in Table 1.A (below).

The admission system crosses natural department boundaries and, hence, requires the removal of traditional organizational barriers and the synchronized involvement of a diversity of players throughout the organization. To orchestrate this effort, a member of the QIC serves as a "champion" for the system. As vice-president over the admissions area, Katrina Van Hoesen serves as champion of this team. The role of the system champion is to guide and coordinate overall system improvement efforts, remove barriers to improvement, allocate resources, serve as a technical resource, and prevent obvious suboptimization.

Clarify current knowledge of the system. Clarification of the admissions system was complicated and time-consuming. It required a great deal of

Table 1.A. The Admission System's Opportunity Statement

The admissions system currently exports chaos and rework throughout the Medical Center, and is dissatisfying to patients, physicians, and internal departments.

The admissions system begins when a test/procedure is scheduled and ends when a patient arrives at the test/procedure site on the day it is to be performed. Improving the admissions system will result in

- reduced rework for the business office and medical records;
- accurate admissions data;
- up-front collections and financial arrangements;
- most patients preadmitted before procedure/visit;
- improved customer satisfaction;
- a more timely admissions process; and
- complete, legible products.

patience and fortitude as well as a willingness to relinquish traditional quick-fix tendencies. A variety of tools were used during the clarification stage to study the flow and interrelationships of the admissions system. Those that we found particularly useful are included in the following examples.

The *process focus worksheet* helped us identify important supplier and customer relationships and answer some key questions about the admissions system: What is it that we produce? Who receives our outputs? What is important to the customers about the outputs they receive? What actions do we perform in order to produce those outputs? What inputs do we need in order to carry out those actions? Who supplies those inputs? What processes are involved in transforming inputs into outputs? This tool (see Table 1.B, below) was very useful for introducing the concept of suppliers and customers to the admissions

Table 1.B. Process Focus Worksheet
Admission System

Supplier	Inputs	Actions	Outputs	Customers	Outcomes
Patient	Patient demo-graphics	Entering • patient demo-graphics • diagnosis	Face	Internal depart-ments	Complete/accurate face sheet
Physician/physician offices	Diagnosis	• authori-zation numbers	Embossed card	Physician offices	Accurate embosser card
Insurance companies	Authori-zation/referral numbers	Calling for verifica-tion/proration informa-tion	Data screens	Third-party payers	Timely de-livery of facesheet/embosser card
Internal depart-ments	Verifi-cation/proration facts	Complet-ing pre-admission question-naires	Patient that has completed all clinical/financial preadmis-sions	Patients	Complete/accurate verification screens Efficient/complete admissions of an AM admit

144270

employees. It offered them a new way to think about what they do on a daily basis. Everyone quickly agreed that without complete and accurate inputs it was impossible to produce a quality product for our customers. Therefore, to make lasting improvements in the admission system we would have to move upstream and work with our key suppliers, especially in the physicians' offices.

A primary purpose of the admissions system is the collection and packaging of data. Patients are suppliers who flow through the admissions system so that data may be collected. The following two tools were used to map out the flow of data and patients.

The *macro product flowchart* was used to portray the key subsystems involved in the collection and flow of data through the admission system. As illustrated in Figure 1.A (below) this flowchart provided a "big picture" and was used to guide more specific clarification and

Figure 1.A. Admissions System: Macro Product Flowchart

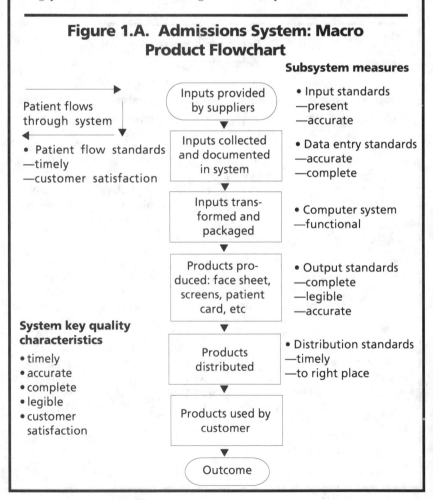

Subsystem measures

Patient flows through system

- Patient flow standards
—timely
—customer satisfaction

System key quality characteristics
- timely
- accurate
- complete
- legible
- customer satisfaction

Inputs provided by suppliers

Inputs collected and documented in system

Inputs trans-formed and packaged

Products pro-duced: face sheet, screens, patient card, etc

Products distributed

Products used by customer

Outcome

- Input standards
—present
—accurate

- Data entry standards
—accurate
—complete

- Computer system
—functional

- Output standards
—complete
—legible
—accurate

- Distribution standards
—timely
—to right place

understanding. Employees in the admissions department then developed detailed flowcharts for each of the subsystems (boxes) represented in the macro product flowchart. Additionally, the macro product flowchart served as a guide for the development of key quality characteristics (KQCs). Via surveys, site visits, and focus groups, we asked the customers of the admissions system what was most important to them about the outputs they received. Their responses were translated into measurable KQCs that can be tracked over time. We are currently tracking the following KQCs: accuracy and completeness of data elements, timeliness of patient flow and data field completion, and patient satisfaction with overall level of service.

The *patient flow matrix* was a useful tool for mapping the flow of patients through the system (see Table 1.C, below). This tool provides a different perspective of the admissions system than the macro product flowchart. We identified eight different types of patient admissions, each with unique flow and processing requirements. To complicate matters, each patient admit type could be further stratified by numerous financial classes, adding additional layers of processing complexity. There was not a standardized admitting process—Parkview's admitting representatives were expected to remember unique processing requirements for all the combinations of admit types and financial classes.

Once we understood the types of patients that were flowing through the admissions system and the sequence of their flow, we further

Table 1.C. Parkview's Admission Department Patient Flow Matrix

	Patient scheduling	Patient presents	Obtain authorization	Patient data fields	Preadmit clinicals	Transportation	Service delivered	Transfer and discharge	Insurance verification	Billing and collections
Same-day surgery	1	2	3	4	5		6	7	8	9
Surgical AM admit (preadmit)		1	2	3	4	5	6	7	8	9
Surgical AM admits	1	2	3	4		5	6	7	8	9
Unplanned admits		1		2		3	4	5	6	7
Outpatient (scheduled)	1	2		3			4			5
Outpatient (unscheduled)		1		2			3			4
Nonpatient admits				1						2

studied patient flow to determine how this flow varied over time, and the length of time patients took to flow through this system (see Figure 1.B, below, for an example of the data collected).

We discovered that we were not handling outpatients, which account for over half of the volume flowing through the admission system, very efficiently. Although outpatients require fewer steps and less processing, they wait in the same queue and go through the same processing line as everybody else. We also identified that patients are spending the majority of their "admission" time waiting in the lobby (an average of ten minutes). Once they are received by the admitting representative, their admission goes relatively quickly (an average of five minutes). Further investigation revealed that the lobby wait times are a function of the two key variables; the number of other patients currently in the system and the availability and accuracy of critical inputs such as diagnosis, insurance card, authorization of procedure, and primary care physician referral.

Perhaps the most interesting and useful information came from the employees who work in the system. Through a visualization and silent brainstorming exercise, we captured the voice of the admissions staff regarding their vision for the admissions department and their thoughts on how and why the current system wasn't meeting our customers' expectations. What emerged from this exercise, in addition to the expected space, equipment, and process problems, was a host of psychosocial issues involving professional identity, teamwork, self-es-

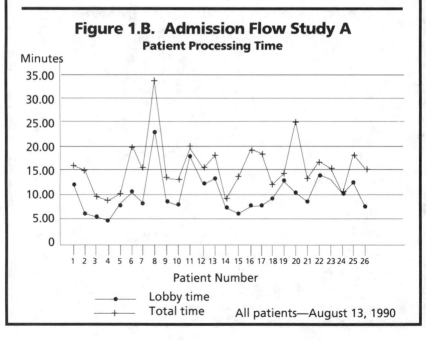

Figure 1.B. Admission Flow Study A
Patient Processing Time

All patients—August 13, 1990

teem, and corporate culture. An affinity/relationship diagram was used to package this information (see Figure 1.C, below).

Understand the causes of system variation. During the "U" phase, data are collected on system KQCs in order to study variation over time. The method of measurement for each KQC of the admission system is as follows:

Figure 1.C. Affinity/Relationship Diagram

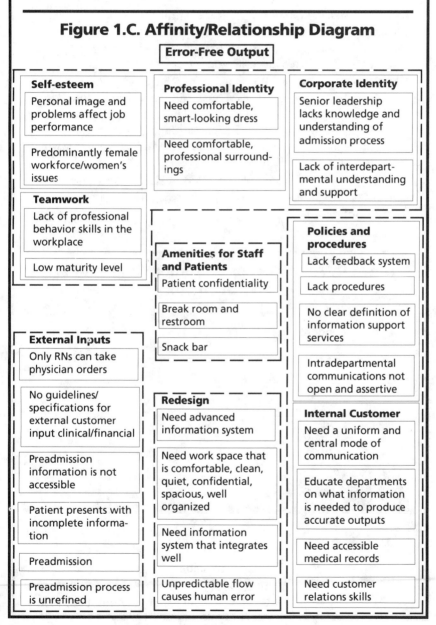

Error-Free Output

Self-esteem
- Personal image and problems affect job performance
- Predominantly female workforce/women's issues

Teamwork
- Lack of professional behavior skills in the workplace
- Low maturity level

Professional Identity
- Need comfortable, smart-looking dress
- Need comfortable, professional surroundings

Corporate Identity
- Senior leadership lacks knowledge and understanding of admission process
- Lack of interdepartmental understanding and support

Amenities for Staff and Patients
- Patient confidentiality
- Break room and restroom
- Snack bar

External Inputs
- Only RNs can take physician orders
- No guidelines/ specifications for external customer input clinical/financial
- Preadmission information is not accessible
- Patient presents with incomplete information
- Preadmission
- Preadmission process is unrefined

Redesign
- Need advanced information system
- Need work space that is comfortable, clean, quiet, confidential, spacious, well organized
- Need information system that integrates well
- Unpredictable flow causes human error

Policies and procedures
- Lack feedback system
- Lack procedures
- No clear definition of information support services
- Intradepartmental communications not open and assertive

Internal Customer
- Need a uniform and central mode of communication
- Educate departments on what information is needed to produce accurate outputs
- Need accessible medical records
- Need customer relations skills

- *Accuracy of data elements.* Admitting representatives collect and plot data on the accuracy of their own data entry work. These data are plotted on a statistical control chart at the workstation over time.
- *Completeness.* The admitting representatives collect information on the completeness of the inputs they receive from their suppliers.
- *Timeliness.* Patient flow studies are conducted biannually to determine patient processing time capabilities. The time it takes to verify a patients' insurance is plotted over time by the verification clerks. They also collect data on the causes for verification delay.
- *Customer satisfaction.* Point-of-service feedback is collected by the admitting representatives. Satisfaction levels are plotted over time, and suggestions for improvement are captured (see Figure 1.D, below). Hospitalwide patient satisfaction surveys also provide data regarding patients' opinions of the admissions system, which can be tracked over time.

Select system improvements. Based on our clarification and understanding of the admissions system, four categories of improvement strategies were initiated:

Figure 1.D. Admissions: Customer Suggestions for Improvement

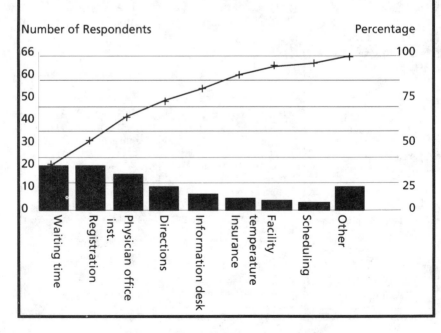

Number of Respondents   Percentage

- *Process improvements.* Several teams were formed to improve specific processes within the admissions system.
- *Innovation and redesign.* System design teams concentrate on building new subsystems or redesigning existing ones. Technological innovation is often a focus of such design teams.
- *Sociocultural interventions.* These interventions include educational and experiential learning focused on self-improvement and teamwork.
- *Management actions.* These improvements do not require formal process improvement teams.

Table 1.D (below) lists all the strategies undertaken within each of these areas.

Table 1.D. System Improvements

Process Improvement Teams
- Emergency room data accuracy team
- Insurance verification team
- Cigna Insurance team
- Patient card delivery team
- Transaction team

System Design and Innovation
- Preadmission system design team
- Scheduling system design team
- Admissions department redesign and renovation

Sociocultural Interventions
- Meyers-Briggs personality assessment
- Professional dress workshop
- Guest speakers at staff meetings
- Ropes course retreat
- Quality improvement education and training
- Communication skills
- Team-building events

Management Actions
- Revise job descriptions
- Upgrade wage scale and position entry requirements
- Flowchart policies and procedures
- Provide additional equipment (printers, headsets, elevated keyboards, file cabinets)
- Redesign forms
- Change data input and display screens in computer system
- Establish a break room for admissions employees
- Require medical terminology certification for all admissions employees

All the process improvement teams directly affect accuracy and timeliness—two of our KQCs. For example, the patient care delivery team was a cross-functional (intradepartmental) team that worked to improve the production and distribution of the patient identification card to the nursing floors and service delivery areas. This process directly impacts the charging, labeling, and charting systems. The transaction team is a functional (within the admissions department) team in which the admitting representatives have improved their own data entry accuracy.

We feel that the most effective improvements will result from the design of a scheduling system and a true preadmissions system, which includes up-front financial counseling and clinical education. It is our vision that when patients are admitted the day of their procedures, they are greeted and taken directly to their rooms or procedure sites.

Summary

Without a doubt, a systems approach has broadened our understanding of the dynamic interrelationships within the admissions system and has guided us in choosing improvement strategies that were previously not obvious. Morale has improved tremendously. The employees in the admissions department understand the processes in which they work and have improved their individual accuracy rates. The amount of rework and chaos exported throughout the hospital has markedly decreased. Customer satisfaction has improved due to higher-quality outputs, better customer service, and the fact that someone is listening to their concerns. We expect that our greatest results will be realized when the new scheduling and preadmissions systems are implemented housewide.

Source: Written and developed by Katrina Van Hoesen, Vice-President Strategic Planning and Marketing, and Donna Wheeler, Director Admissions. Reprinted with permission from Parkview Episcopal Medical Center, Pueblo, Colorado, 1991

(continued from page 23)
necessary resources, remove barriers, and provide progress reports to the QIC and board.

All teams use HCA's FOCUS-PDCA process improvement methodology (see Figure 1.4, pages 34–35) as well as meeting management techniques and the quality control tools (see Appendix A, page 255). The use of FOCUS-PDCA and the emphasis on data collection have been crucial to the success of recent team efforts. A structured process provides guidelines for teams to follow and helps team members focus on the process being investigated rather than their own personal agenda. A team leader who is also the "owner" of the process heads each team, and a facilitator is assigned. Table 1.3 (pages 36–37) lists many of Parkview's team activities.

All teams at Parkview communicate and report their activities and results in several ways. Storyboards are used to display team findings and are organized according to the steps that make up the FOCUS-PDCA cycle. Teams hang their storyboards on the walls for staff to view and use them to give presentations on their activities. Teams take turns presenting their activities at the Quality Forum conducted by the QIC each month. The forum provides an opportunity for the QIC to give helpful feedback to the teams. On these occasions, Pugh and other members of the QIC offer words of encouragement and advice on the direction the team might take. The forum also allows teams to communicate to the QIC their needs for additional resources or assistance.

QA/QI Relationship

Rather than discard all elements of QA as meaningless, staff at Parkview hope to improve the Joint Commission's ten-step monitoring and evaluation process by integrating it with FOCUS-PDCA. This involves more than just using QI tools for QA activities and displaying data. The nursing service has developed a careful, step-by-step cross-walk of the two processes that establishes equivalencies at each step. This integration is being attempted not only to reduce the barriers inherent in the language, philosophy, and tools, but to identify the elements of QA and QI that are valuable and amenable to integration.

The medical staff office continues to conduct the medical staff monitoring functions required by the Joint Commission (for example, surgical case review, blood usage evaluation). A project currently underway in blood usage evaluation is yielding good results in improving communication among prescribing physicians and the blood bank. Also, the medical staff services monitors a number of generic indicators, such as death, returns to surgery, and so forth that might identify issues for teams to evaluate.

While there are still some aspects of the present Joint Commission standards for QA that Parkview hopes will be revised in the future to make them more compatible with their QI efforts, they have succeeded in effective integration.

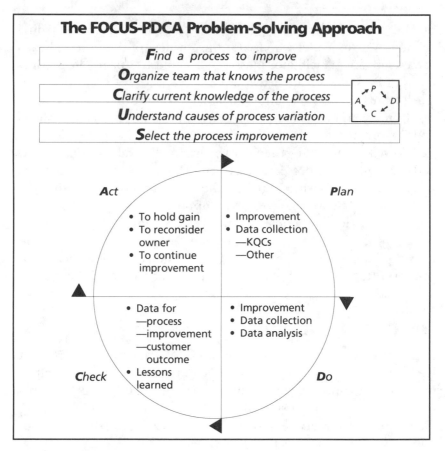

The FOCUS-PDCA Problem-Solving Approach

Find a process to improve
Organize team that knows the process
Clarify current knowledge of the process
Understand causes of process variation
Select the process improvement

Act

- To hold gain
- To reconsider owner
- To continue improvement

Plan

- Improvement
- Data collection
  —KQCs
  —Other

Check

- Data for
  —process
  —improvement
  —customer outcome
- Lessons learned

Do

- Improvement
- Data collection
- Data analysis

Education

Pugh estimates that Parkview spent less than $100,000 in the first year for outside assistance and education. QI training began with senior management and the board and has been cascaded down the organization. As of May 1991, all department managers have been trained in QI concepts, including statistics and team skills, and approximately 450–500 employees have received a quality awareness class. Facilitators provide "just-in-time" tool training to teams. Important in the success of Parkview's training program is that leaders and managers become trainers themselves once they are trained. For example, Pugh and other members of the QIC teach quality awareness classes, and department managers teach their staff QI methods and tools as part of their departmental rollouts. Parkview also emphasizes self-learning: Senior management and department heads take time out of their meetings to discuss journal articles or books related to QI, and senior

The FOCUS-PDCA Problem-Solving Approach (continued)

Find an opportunity	Organize the team	Clarify the process	Understand the variation(s)	Select an Improvement
• Who is the customer? • What is the name of the process? • What are the process boundaries? • Is the opportunity statement there? • Is it clear? • Who will benefit from the improvement? • How is the process tied to the hospital as a system?	• Is the team size appropriate? • Do the members represent people who work in the process? • Has the owner of the process been identified? • Does the team's knowledge of the process align with the boundaries in the opportunity statement? • What is the team's name?	• Is the process presented at a level of detail that identifies possible causes of variation? • Is there evidence of agreement on a best method as represented by a single flow chart? • Do the boundaries of the flow chart align with the opportunity statement and the team? • After reaching consensus, were obvious improvements made in this phase? • Did the team defer any improvements to the "Select" phase? • Is there evidence that the "actual" flow of the process was documented rather than some perceived flow?	• How did the team identify the KQC (key quality characteristic) and potential KPVs (key process variables)? • Is there an operational definition for the KQC and the potential KPV? • Is there a data collection plan? Is it clear how the data will be collected? Who will collect it? • Does the team understand how long it will take to collect enough data to make a decision? • How does the performance of the process vary over time? • Can the team show a relationship between KQC and the KPV?	• How did the team select the improvement? • Are there any data or other evidence to support the selection? • What were the criteria for making the decision?

Plan
- Does the team have a plan for piloting the improvement and collecting it?
- Does the pilot plan indicate dates, communications, and ownership of specific steps?
- What training is necessary?

Do
- How was the plan executed?
- Did any contingencies arise?
- Were dates on the data collection plan met?

Act
- Did the team act to implement the process gain beyond the pilot?
- Did the team act to generalize the lessons learned from the pilot? Or did the team act to discard the planned improvement?
- Can the team find another opportunity for improvement within this process?
- What did the team learn from the effort?

Check
- Do the data on the run chart suggest that the process changed?
- How did the data change?
- Does the team know anything that helps explain any evident change?
- Is the team comfortable that enough data are present to support an action?
- If the team is not comfortable with the amount of data or the knowledge provided by the data, what is the plan for obtaining more?

Roadmap
- Does the roadmap indicate key actions that the team is likely to take?
- What is the time frame?
- Is the team on track?
- Is there evidence of updating or reviewing the roadmap?
- Where is the team on the roadmap?

Source: Reprinted with permission from HCA Quality Resource Group, Nashville, Tennessee, 1991.

Figure 1.4. Parkview has adapted the FOCUS-PDCA problem-solving approach.

35

Table 1.3. A Sample of Parkview's Team Activities

IV QIT. This team was initiated by a nursing department director at the urging of her staff to look at the process of IV administration on the medical floor. This team has begun identifying causes of variation in IV administration and has begun standardizing the process of starting, maintaining, and discontinuing IVs.

Cardiac Surgery Intensive Care Unit Admission QIT. This team standardized the process of admitting new postoperative cardiac surgery patients to the intensive care unit. Led and initiated by the intensive care unit department manager, the team reduced the amount of time required to admit a patient to the unit from an average time of 20 minutes to under 8 minutes. In addition, the team began working with the operating room and anesthesiologists to standardize IV lines and reduce costs.

Recycling Team. As a result of a suggestion by employees to begin a recycling program, senior management organized a recycling team to develop a process of recycling paper and other recyclable materials. As a result of their efforts, the team designed a process that resulted in a negligible incremental cost and a reduction of solid waste removal and landfill fees by over $10,000 per year.

Operating Room Charge QIT. As a spin-off to the charging system efforts, the operating room charge team completely redesigned the process for charging in the operating room. Their improvement resulted in eliminating an estimated $2,500 per month in lost operating room charges.

Patient Chart QIT. As a spin-off to the clinical results reporting system, a nursing team has looked at the process of assembling and maintaining the patient's chart. The team has currently developed a standardized approach to be used hospitalwide and a check-and-act mechanism to ensure that patient chart assembly remains standardized.

Home Care Billing Team. A team of business office and home care employees worked together to improve the home care billing process, resulting in reduction of home care billing errors from over 100% of all bills to less than 1%.

Medical Staff Services QIT. The medical staff services team worked with a committee of the board and medical staff to clarify and flowchart the critical processes of medical staff application, reappointment, and disciplinary action. As a result of standardizing the process, the members of the Credentials and Board Committees reviewing the application can focus on the credentials of the applicant rather than problems in the credentialing process itself.

Table 1.3. A Sample of Parkview's Team Activities (continued)

Invalid Outpatient Diagnosis QIT. When the medical records and admissions departments formed this team, they chose to focus on supplying a valid outpatient diagnosis from the point the patient information is collected to the point the record is coded. The first data showed a 13% invalid outpatient diagnosis rate. Current data following process improvements show a 4% rate, thus decreasing the amount of rework and chaos exported throughout the hospital.

Pediatric Menu QIT. After watching pediatric patients throwing away food, the pediatric and dietary units formed a team to improve the pediatric menu process. Data showed a 50% food eaten rate. A menu revision was suggested, planned, and implemented, resulting in 89% food eaten.

Tray Delivery QIT. This team is in its final "Act" phase of the PDCA cycle. It led to the reduction of undelivered trays from 40% to 5% housewide. This is a tremendous cost/productivity improvement as well as a start to meeting customer expectations of a timely hot or cold meal.

Socio-Cultural System Team. This team tackled the sociocultural aspect of interpersonal and working relationships within a natural work group. An affinity diagram and force field analysis was developed that showed internal and external issues as well as the barriers to a team culture. The team suggested a team-building workshop for employee groups. The team is in the "Do" phase and will regather data to determine effectiveness of the improvement cycle.

First Case QIT. This was the first team that involved both medical staff and other hospital staff. They used the scientific method to reduce late starts in the operating room from 180 minutes late per month to starting an average of 1.61 minutes early, thus saving staff costs and maximizing room productivity and delighting physicians.

Source: *Reprinted with permission from Parkview Episcopal Medical Center, Pueblo, Colorado, 1991.*

---

and middle management are expected to devise their own personal QI learning plans.

Parkview has developed their own quality awareness course as well as a facilitator training course, which recently graduated its first class of facilitators. The QI coach is instrumental in the development of course curriculums; Ivey receives resources and assistance from Quorum, Parkview's management company. An outside consultant, Marcus

Padgett, was hired as well to provide training in statistical process control and theory.

QI Supports

Customer-supplier feedback mechanisms. All QI efforts at Parkview, both on the organizationwide and department level, tie back to the identification of customers and their needs. Key processes that impact these customers (for example, dietary) and key quality characteristics of those processes (for example, delivery of food) are identified. Once the key quality characteristics of a process are determined, staff determine the key process variables for measuring the quality of those processes (for example, time, temperature, cost).

Formal feedback from patients, employees, and physicians is sought mainly through the hospital quality trend (HQT) survey, which was developed for HCA and Quorum by NDP Research in Nashville, Tennessee. Results of the HQT survey provide macro patient feedback on key hospital services. Since many Quorum hospitals use the HQT survey, Parkview can compare its results with those of other hospitals. Another feedback mechanism is the SRI/Gallup survey of the hospital, which provides information on the community health care preferences. The hospital is also asking the question "what is the main thing we can do better?" in admissions, housekeeping, and dietary and is using the results to identify process improvement opportunities.

One strong indicator of customer satisfaction at Parkview is what staff refer to as "customer murmurs." All staff are encouraged to pay close attention to the "grumblings" of patients, physicians, and others. Medical records even began a log book of these murmurs and developed Pareto charts to graphically display the results.

Management information systems. Although Parkview has three data systems that provide access to financial, clinical, and ordering data, these data systems have not yet been integrated. Most process-oriented data needed for QI efforts are collected by hand. For instance, the radiology team, addressing turnaround of radiographic reports, hand tallies the arrival times of patients. Parkview's experience has been that the most effective data collection is by employees on the processes that they work with as part of their daily work lives. "Process improvement at the employee level is the fundamental building block of continuous improvement," Pugh says. Most of the data collection at this level will continue to be done by hand.

Staff are continually learning how to simplify data collection methods, focusing on the important data versus extraneous data that are often collected out of habit. In many areas, employees collect data by plotting the next point on a graph on a real-time basis instead of collecting vast amounts of data and giving it to the department managers to sort out. "The major misconception is that information systems are a 'silver bullet' for QI," Pugh says. "Hospital information systems can and do help us identify where to focus our efforts [that is, which processes to work on] and are helpful in judging the macro effect of our many improvements."

Parkview is in the process of installing MedisGroups, which will provide judgments on the severity of illness both pretreatment and posttreatment. The systems are useful for helping the hospital identify opportunities for improvement and prioritizing those opportunities.

Reward and recognition. After attending HCA's QI courses, Dorothy Gill, vice-president for human resources, concurred with Deming's views that performance evaluations emphasize individual accomplishment over teamwork and formed a team to address the issue. Salary increases at Parkview had traditionally been tied directly with performance evaluations. After extensively researching performance feedback practices at other organizations and in the literature and reviewing the complexity and variation within Parkview's process, the team developed an approach that did away with its traditional merit rating system and instituted a policy that employees would receive performance reviews on their anniversary date. Across-the-board salary increases were given on the same date each year, based on environmental factors such as inflation, comparable increases in other organizations, and what the hospital could afford. The team polled staff on the new system. Results showed that the changes were received positively but further improvement was necessary. Employees scored the change more positively than department managers.

In August 1991, the hospital took the next step in implementing Deming's philosophy and abolished the traditional annual performance appraisal system in response to employees' remarks. The performance appraisal is being replaced with annual review of employee educational and training needs, job description, and periodic skills assessments. It is anticipated that the average department manager will save over 80 hours per year on paperwork associated with performance appraisals. One major issue that has not been resolved is how to financially recognize the excellent individual performer.

Gill is working with representatives from several other Quorum hospitals on a new approach to performance feedback based on the

PDCA cycle. According to Gill, the team's objective is to develop a guide for managers and employees that will facilitate two-way communication concerning the individual's development as a whole person, identification of barriers to pride of workmanship (that is, equipment, training, relationships), and customer feedback.

To reward the accomplishments of teams, Parkview throws an annual Quality Day Celebration. People from across the country are invited to visit Parkview and see presentations by QI teams. In 1990 more than 50 visitors attended. The hospital also reports on team activities through their monthly newsletter, *The Quality News*, and publishes an annual report of all department QI activities. A more immediate reward structure for teams is the monthly Quality Forum described in "QI Process."

Benchmarking. Although Pugh wants to be able to gauge where Parkview is in terms of QI, he is uncertain if health care has reached the point at which benchmarking would provide useful feedback. He cites several reasons:

- Hospitals do not yet have the data needed for accurate comparison;
- Many of the systems Parkview would want to compare itself with are mediocre;
- Parkview is not yet certain what to benchmark itself against;
- There are more providers in health care than in industry (that is, it is simpler for Xerox to compare itself against the handful of other copier makers than for a hospital to compare itself against the thousands of other hospitals); and
- Benchmarking is not philosophically consistent with Deming's ideas of continuous improvement.

However, Pugh admits, "we can't know where we are until we look at others." Parkview uses the HQT surveys from Quorum as its primary benchmarking source. Staff have also begun comparing themselves against industry (for example, billing processes).

Physician Involvement

At the beginning of the QI efforts, the QIC decided to wait to involve physicians extensively. Management did not want to mobilize the medical staff before they were sure QI methods would be successful. The approach to clinical QI was not certain; it was much easier to make the connection from industrial QI examples to hospital operational functions than to the clinical arena. Management also did not want clinicians initially confusing QI efforts with traditional QA, which focuses on finding what the clinician is doing wrong rather than what is wrong with the process.

During the first years of QI, senior management "decided to treat physicians more as customers than as suppliers in the rollout of QI," Pugh says. They formed teams to investigate processes that physicians owned or controlled or that they found particularly burdensome. That is why clinical results reporting and admissions were chosen as two key areas of focus. These successes piqued physicians' curiosities and laid the groundwork for Parkview to begin moving QI into the clinical sphere.

Parkview's rollout plan emphasizes the initial education of physicians, including the following:

- Developing basic QI physician courses by Pugh and the vice-president, medical staff services;
- Incorporating the QI meeting format into medical staff meetings; and
- Including physicians on hospital teams.

Recently, a new position, medical director of clinical quality improvement, was created to assist in the rollout of QI into the clinical area and lead the integration of QI in the medical staff processes. In this role, Keith Wilson, MD, chairs the Quality and Utilization Review Committee of the Medical Staff, on which each clinical department is represented. Wilson will also be working with the patient delivery system champions.

Conclusion

As illustrated throughout this chapter, QI at Parkview is focused by the leaders, taught and championed by the leaders, structured by the leaders, and rewarded by the leaders. It is this focus and direction that empowers staff to creatively approach problems and opportunities for improvement. Staff own one vital component—the data. It is the data "that set you free," Pugh says. As Renay Hammond, admissions clerk says, data provide proof on paper. "We [in admissions] get a lot more respect than we used to. Because they [others in hospital] have started to see data on all the work we do down here.

2 Coloring Outside the Lines
USAF Medical Center, Wright-Patterson Dayton, Ohio

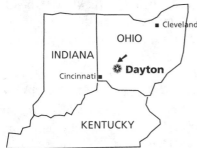

Type of hospital: Air Force medical center
Scope of services: General medical/surgical
Beds: 301, with an average census of 220
Extent of TQM involvement: The hospital began TQM efforts in 1988. Strengths are in the buy in and rollout of TQM methods and concepts throughout all levels of the organization, including physicians, as revealed by the successes of teams and other activities. Strategic planning is in the initial stages

Special aspects of Wright-Patterson's TQM activities:
— Began movement in environment already promoting TQM
— Staff are "coloring" outside traditionally stringent lines to improve the provision of care
— Physician involvement from beginning
— Strong Quality Council, which was tested by a change of leaders mid stream into their TQM effort
— Bob's Bucket Theory
— Approach to QA/QI

Ask staff at Wright-Patterson Medical Center (WPMC) when they knew management was serious about total quality management (TQM), and they recall the expression on the Air Force inspector general's face two years ago when the entire medical center turned out with noisemakers to cheer both the unsatisfactory and satisfactory ratings

43

they received. The commander at the time, Colonel Charles Roadman, had introduced the hospital to TQM the year before. He recognized the hospital would receive unsatisfactory ratings in certain areas but decided against fixing the problems in a suboptimal manner just to do well on the survey. Instead he told the inspector general that the problems at WPMC were process-related or the result of budgetary constraints and asked all staff to turn up at the hospital auditorium for the inspector's closing report and "celebrate" all the ratings they received. "The inspector thought he'd put up the wrong rating," said OB Murray, director of managed health care, remembering the cheers and noise raised over the first unsatisfactory rating. That day an important message was sent throughout the medical center; staff left the auditorium less afraid to make mistakes and understanding that everyone at WPMC, from physicians to admissions clerks, owned and contributed to the medical center's success.

The inspector general was not the first or last to walk away from WPMC dumbfounded. Contrary to the stereotypical image of a military facility, civil disobedience is encouraged at WPMC when it means quality improvement. Members of the Quality Council jokingly refer to their tactics as "bureaucratic terrorism." Major Sandy Murray, director of TQM, emphasizes that bureaucratic terrorism involves understanding the bureaucracy well enough to change it. "We haven't had to throw any grenades yet," she said, "but we are terrorists in the sense that we challenge the status quo." Colonel Kitty Taylor, director of nursing, emphasizes that staff at WPMC are continually "coloring outside the lines." Staff from top to bottom are encouraged to question procedures that are "non–value-added." The hospital has asked for numerous waivers from procedures when staff discover they can do something better, including posting unnecessary lab results, record review, and meeting minutes. In the first six months of their "help sheet" suggestion program, 125 ideas for improving existing procedures were submitted by staff, resulting in an estimated savings of $100,000. At Quality Council meetings, military rank essentially disappears and opinions fly across the table. Decisions are not approved until each member sticks his or her thumb up (approval). A thumb that is parallel to the table is not a positive or negative vote but forces additional discussion in order to try to reach consensus. This leads to "ownership by the group of the decision," said Colonel Terence Cunningham, administrator. No person's opinion carries more weight than another's, and yet there remains a deep respect for rank and regulation. Members of the Quality Council still rise when the present commander, Colonel John Anderson, MD, enters the room, and regulations are followed unless a waiver is obtained.

Description and Demographics

Innovation is part of the historical character of WPMC. In 1904, Orville Wright, knowing there must be a better way to travel, flew over Huffman Prairie for five minutes and four seconds. Aviation research and development continued to flourish in Dayton after the Wright brothers. Several large flying fields were established including Wilbur Wright Field, renamed Patterson Field in 1931 after Lt Frank Patterson crashed while flight testing the synchronization of a machine gun and propeller. After World War II, the various fields became one installation—Wright-Patterson Air Force Base, which is one of six bases in the Air Force Logistics Command (AFLC). The AFLC, headquartered at Wright-Patterson Air Force Base, is responsible for buying, supplying, transporting, and maintaining everything needed to keep Air Force weapon systems operationally ready. While WPMC is located at Wright-Patterson Air Force Base, the Air Force treats the medical center as a separate organization because of its size. The medical center has a dotted-line relationship with the base command, and Anderson reports directly to the AFLC commander.

WPMC provides care for military staff at Wright-Patterson Air Force Base, as well as their dependents, retired military, and dependents of retired military. The hospital's boundaries go far beyond the Dayton area or even the state of Ohio; WPMC is also the tertiary referral facility for Department of Defense Region VI, which includes ten states. The local beneficiary population is estimated at 60,861, and an estimated 900,000 potential patients within the Department of Defense region can receive care at WPMC as well.

WPMC is better described as a "health city than a hospital," according to Cunningham. A 301-bed facility, WPMC is the second largest hospital in the Air Force when measured by total inpatient and outpatient work load. There were nearly 60,000 inpatient visits and approximately 600,000 outpatient visits in fiscal year 1990. Over 70 specialties and subspecialties are provided. WPMC is affiliated with the local Wright State University School of Medicine. Graduate medical education programs are offered and residencies provided for approximately 100 physicians and student-physicians. Nursing education and residencies/internships in hospital administration and psychology are provided as well.

WPMC had an early advantage in moving toward TQM; the medical center began TQM in an environment already promoting it. Early in 1988 the AFLC decided to move toward TQM and began exposing senior officers to the experiences of Xerox, Ford, and other industry leaders. Being a military hospital, WPMC has been able to take advantage of many resources the Air Force offers, including the courses in TQM and statistical process control provided by the Air Force Institute of Technology (AFIT) located with the Medical Center at Wright-Patterson Air Force Base. As discussed in "Education," WPMC has an agreement with AFIT, which is a component of the Air University. The Logistic Command's TQM efforts were rewarded recently when it won the President's Award in 1991. This award, the military equivalent of the Malcolm Baldrige Award in the civilian sector, recognizes great progress in quality; WPMC's activities were instrumental in the Command's successful effort. Cunningham says the process of preparing the application, not so much winning the award, helped accelerate the rollout, emphasize statistical thinking, and deploy the TQM message throughout the organization.

History

The speed with which TQM took root at WPMC is linked directly to the sense of crisis that hung over the hospital when Roadman took command. A seven-year, $123-million construction project had seriously disturbed access to the hospital. Census dropped to 120 patients, and all mental health and pediatrics patients had to be referred elsewhere. When Anderson visited the hospital in connection with the inspector general's office, prior to Roadman's assumption of command, the place was "an absolute disaster." Staff realized they were trying to function in a system that did not work; it was either change or not survive. "The sense of crisis was very real," S. Murray remembers. "Roadman didn't want to go to dinner parties because people barraged him" with complaints about not being able to get an appointment for an outpatient visit.

"Staff compared the pre-TQM atmosphere at WPMC to a medieval fiefdom," says Lieutenant Colonel D'Aquila-Lloyd, director, clinical quality services. Lieutenant Colonel Bob Murray, associate administrator, describes it as "a series of fiefdoms connected by a central heating and air conditioning system." The hospital was organized by medical departments, and each physician department head was primarily interested in the strength of his or her own department. "Prior to 1988 my job in pediatrics was to get an 'A' in our department's accreditation report," said Colonel Jerry Foster, chairman of the department of pediatrics and acting director of hospital services. "I didn't care what surgery or other departments got."

Roadman arrived at the hospital, immediately became exposed to TQM at the Logistics Command Headquarters, and began orienting staff to the principles of customer-and-supplier relationships and statistical process control. He helped staff see the "picture of fiefdoms," according to Chief Master Sergeant Ken Vandegrift, senior enlisted advisor. Roadman provided the impetus WPMC needed to make a cultural change. "We needed someone to ride in on a white horse and say at first, 'you guys are responsible for running this place as a team,'" Taylor said.

If placed in a run chart, WPMC's TQM activities would not climb drastically until late 1990. Team members easily pinpoint the date their team's activities began taking off—the same day they received extensive training and were given a standardized approach to problem solving. Until 1990 staff studied various approaches and piloted TQM methods and concepts in the hospital but had no clear sense of direction. Looking back, senior management dubbed 1989 as the year of "uninformed optimism." "We thought we'd solve all our problems with fast PATs [process action teams] and would have a solution in two hours or two weeks," Cunningham said. But the initial PATs "failed miserably." That first stage of learning and reevaluation was vitally important, however, in developing a culture at WPMC that was strong enough to withstand a leadership change. Several key events led to this paradigm shift:

- Roadman started a reading club for senior management, called the Upton Society, to review TQM literature and discuss how they could initiate TQM at the hospital. Senior staff and department heads began to attend TQM courses locally and across the country.

- Other clubs formed, including one made up of heads of the medical staff departments, informally referred to as the "bull walruses," who met over breakfast. "At first, nobody even wanted to reach for the doughnuts," Foster said. But once they started discussing each other's needs "the fiefdoms saw something for themselves."

- A growing interest in customer opinion led staff to interview patients in the hospital and outside the base exchange and commissary. When the same survey was later administered to staff, the results differed drastically. Staff identified technical outcome as the important concern while patients responded that access to the medical center was their main desire. "In terms of technical outcomes we were doing great," Vandegrift said. "But there was no . . . access."

- The first management "off-site" meetings were held to discuss the hospital's vision and strategy, and the executive staff decided to focus on the problem of access across the hospital.

- The Quality Council was formed to oversee the rollout of TQM, and a part-time TQM director (also referred to as the QI coach), who would later become full-time, was appointed. The Council, which handles the hospital's operational functions, is made up largely of the same senior management who serve on the executive committee, the patient relations coordinator, senior civilian, and a noncommissioned officer.

A key structural change occurred in 1989 that helped align the organization with TQM. Until then, WPMC was organized along discipline lines or "stovepipes" (for example, all nurses reported to the director of nursing), which discouraged collaboration and encouraged the fiefdoms to flourish. Recognizing that they were floundering in the current structure, department heads initiated the move to matrix management in the winter of 1989. Matrix teams were formed within each major clinical service to break down the stovepipes and provide for cross-disciplinary management of patient care units. The teams consisted of a physician-clinician department chairman, administrator, and superintendent (that is, senior enlisted personnel) and senior nurse. One of the more representative and successful matrix teams is the obstetrics and gynecology matrix. This team smooths the passages that a typical obstetric patient faces, from pregnancy testing to lab and imaging services, from prenatal clinic care to inpatient care including birth registration, from newborn care to postpartum follow-up.

When Roadman was reassigned in 1990, the executive staff feared the inroads they had made might have been in vain. But the TQM philosophy was so deeply ingrained in senior management at that point that they rose to meet the challenge. Anderson tells how he received a series of phone calls from executive staff at the medical center before he arrived as the new commander. They informed him that WPMC was a TQM organization and hoped he would command using the same methods. "I was fascinated," Anderson said. He did not know a lot about TQM at the time. However, he recognized that he needed to "run ahead of the pack" if he wanted a pack to lead. Senior management members agree that the change of commands came at a key point; the different personalities of the two leaders helped them make the transition to TQM. With his hard-charging style, Roadman had challenged staff and gotten senior management to take their first steps toward the transition. Anderson, with a very collaborative style, has helped staff continue to make this transition in "walking the talk and walking the walk" and to accomplish things as a team.

Within this collaborative culture, the Quality Council began re-evaluating their TQM activities and recognized that staff needed more training and structure. In 1990, the year they titled "informed pessimism," members of the Quality Council began meeting bimonthly and taking a more aggressive role in the rollout of TQM. The Quality Council adopted Quorum's rollout plan (see page 108 of Chapter 4) and modified it to their own time frames. They also began training staff in the FOCUS-PDCA process improvement approach (see pages 34–35 of Chapter 1). The part-time QI coach became a full-time position, and S. Murray was provided with an assistant. Her office is primarily charged with developing and teaching TQM curriculum to staff, providing support to the Quality Council and PAT teams, tracking the training being accomplished, and serving as an in-house consultant on TQM methods and tools. S. Murray compares her position to an octopus with its many different arms. Her office reaches out to and provides support in TQM to the different levels of the hospital. Eventually, Murray sees her job disappearing. As the concepts and tools become more and more ingrained in the organization, she doesn't feel there will be need for a QI coach.

Staff at WPMC moved quickly from "uninformed optimism" to "informed pessimism." Midway into 1991 they are moving toward their vision of a TQM organization. Executive staff demonstrate the concepts in daily activities, departments are actively identifying customers and suppliers, and quality assurance (QA) activities have changed drastically. As explained in "Strategy," the executive staff are now devising the strategy that will drive and maintain this enthusiasm for TQM.

Philosophy

WPMC is not working to become WPMC + TQM but rather WPMC$_2$—

an entirely different organization. The hospital is redirecting all its activities in terms of TQM. "TQM is not a panacea," Anderson said, "but an effective management model." To emphasize this philosophy, senior management have incorporated TQM into their vision: "...The Medical Center is ready to deal with a rapidly changing environment using principles of total quality management...." The medical center's executive staff learned quickly, under Roadman's tutelage, that quality medical care is more than just technical outcome. It also includes cost and scheduling (a term used to describe some of the service components of health care such as access, courtesy, and sensitivity). This notion of three parameters of quality has been incorporated in the center's vision statement: "...to deliver reasonably priced, state-of-the-art medicine and service to meet the needs of the patient population...." They defined five organizational values that support their vision: professionalism, teamwork, customer focus, employee focus, and continuous improvement. Executive staff have shared the vision with all members of the medical center via briefings in individual work centers at different times of the day and night, which are convenient to the personnel on duty. The hospital demonstrates its commitment to its vision by adhering to the following principles:

- The primary focus of quality is the customer, both internal and external;

- Necessary top-down commitment of executive staff to TQM, including teaching of TQM;

- Empowerment of staff to continuously improve the processes they work with;

- Commitment of resources up front; and

- Recognition of the importance of continually training.

As military personnel, staff try to correlate their management approach with the values and principles of the armed forces. "Professionalism" is one of their organizational values, and staff strive to embody "the dual cultural values of the health care profession and the profession of arms." Contrary to the stereotypical image of a military organization, however, their values also "encourage risk taking and creative thinking." As already highlighted, staff take pride at WPMC in coloring outside the lines and have saved significant costs by looking beyond policies to find better ways to do things. Anderson admits this is "a radical departure for the Air Force." But staff at WPMC show no conflict between TQM and following orders. While staff challenge the status quo, it is "not done with disrespect but with data and rationale,"

S. Murray said. These are the same principles endorsed by TQM—solutions are arrived at through data and an understanding of the larger picture.

Strategy

Bob Murray devised "Bob's Bucket Theory" after witnessing the manner in which TQM spread through the medical center. According to Quorum's rollout plan (page 108), an organization should complete each step or "bucket" from the top down before moving on to the next step (that is, fill the top leadership "bucket" before beginning the middle leadership "bucket"). In reality, Lt Colonel Murray maintains the rollout of TQM is not systematic. Enthusiasm spreads more like a "firehose effect," Murray said. "The force and volume is so great, buckets are being filled up at different amounts and different levels" throughout WPMC. A "tremendous grass-roots movement" has developed in some departments and their "buckets" are already half full. Rather than put the brakes on this enthusiasm by making staff wait until senior management has finalized the organization's TQM strategy, the medical center has decided to let TQM flow through the organization at its natural speed. "It makes more work for management" (for example, keeping up with resource demands), but capturing the "excitement of staff makes it worth it," Anderson said.

As buckets fill at different speeds throughout WPMC, senior management are busy filling the bucket that deals with planning. The Quality Council (which includes all those on the Executive Committee) and selected key staff members presently meet eight times a year (quarterly three-day planning "off-sites" and a one-day meeting between each off-site) to develop objectives that the entire organization will focus on and indicators that will allow staff to measure the hospital's success. WPMC is developing a customer-focused strategic plan, based on the Florida Power and Light concepts presented at the medical center by Dr Haudiberg, former chief executive officer of Florida Power and Light. As illustrated in Figure 2.1 (page 52) this formulaic model assists staff in developing measurable strategic objectives for the organization as a whole and for each individual department.

To arrive at organizationwide objectives, the Executive Committee began with the medical center's mission, which has five elements:

- providing and arranging for comprehensive quality community health care services;

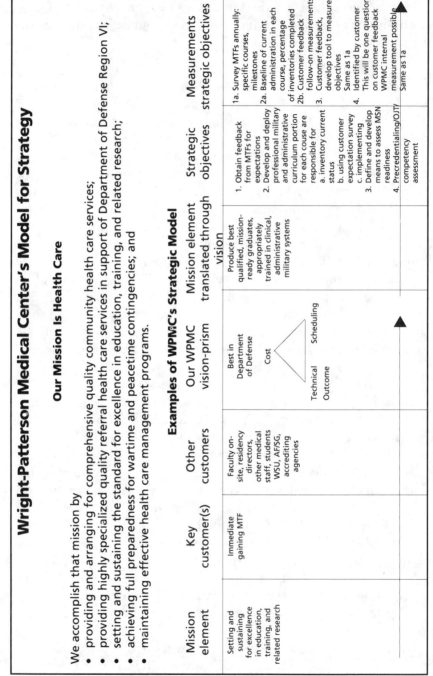

Figure 2.1. To determine strategic objectives, both organizationwide and at the department level, staff plug each of the five elements of WPMC's mission into the formulaic model illustrated above.

- providing highly specialized quality referral health care services in support of Department of Defense Region VI;
- setting and sustaining the standard for excellence in education, training, and related research;
- achieving full preparedness for war and peacetime contingencies; and
- maintaining effective health care management programs.

For each of these five elements, the committee considered key customers, other customers, and WPMC's vision (as expressed by the prism of cost, scheduling, and technical outcome) before arriving at a strategic vision, strategic objectives, and measurements for achieving each mission element. Figure 2.1 provides an example of strategic objectives and measurements for one of the five mission elements. Each department will use this same formula to develop department objectives that are linked with the hospital's mission.

The Quality Council recognized the need to build a critical mass of staff educated in TQM to address the high turnover rate in the military. The Quality Council determined the best way to accomplish this was to deploy TQM at the department level. In addition to the training of key staff department by department (see "Education"), each department is also beginning to analyze its customers and the important processes—an activity called departmental task analysis. Some departments are further along than others. Major Ralph Charlip, director of the aerovac department describes how TQM has become part of his job. (Aerovac or aeromedical evacuation is the movement of patients from one installation to another for specialized care by means of various types of medically equipped aircraft.) A group from all departments involved plotted on a flowchart the process of arrival time updates of inbound aerovac flights. A communication problem was identified in the notification chain. As a result of interaction, vast improvements were made to appropriately accommodate the customer. Matrix management has also helped deploy TQM thinking throughout the departments involved. By working in teams that cross disciplines, staff better understand the concepts of systems and customers.

Staff throughout WPMC acknowledge that TQM has affected their roles in the organization. According to B. Murray, the "people who stand to benefit the most [from TQM] are the oppressed, such as nursing [staff]." He believes some administrators will "see themselves as losers." Management has to realize that "the way to gain power is to give it away," Murray said. The deployment of TQM is often difficult for department heads and middle managers according to Anderson because they are "battered from two directions." They are pressured by their subordinates as well as senior management. One department head said that it becomes "hard to say no to people. TQM creates a yes, yes, yes environment." He stressed the importance of determining "what battles to pick and fight," otherwise resources will be diverted in too many directions.

QI Process

Staff throughout WPMC have begun using TQM methods and tools in their day-to-day activities. Involvement in PATs has helped expose staff to these concepts and has provided an excellent environment to attack a problem. WPMC has over a dozen PATs currently investigating processes across the organization. (See Table 2.1, below, for a sample

---

Table 2.1. A Sample of WPMC's PAT Activities

Nutritional Medicine/Nursing PAT. Improve regular selective menu delivery return system. Desire to improve return rate of food from 40% to 75% and reduce wasted food and patient complaints that they did not receive food they ordered.

Consultation System PAT. Improve outpatient physician consultation system by simplifying procedures, resulting in shortened consultation time, reductions in misplaced consultation forms and improved feedback to provider, patient, and consultant.

Surgery Scheduling PAT. Improve surgery scheduling to increase utilization of surgery suite. Specifically, the team is working to reduce surgery cancellations and turnover time between cases and to improve the scheduling process.

Convalescent Leave/Subsisting Elsewhere PAT. Evaluate process used to grant military patients convalescence leave to reduce patient records and reduce confusion for patients and staff.

Inpatient Medication Management PAT. Improve process of ordering and delivering of IV admixtures to reduce current level of IVs and ensure highest possible patient care. (See the case study on pages 57–63 for more on this PAT.)

Physical Exam PAT. Improve scheduling and processing of physical exams of aircrew members to decrease completion time error rate and to avoid grounding of aircrews.

Patient Transfer PAT. Improve communications of a patient transfer between nursing units to all support services. The process begins with

---

of these activities.) To prove their commitment to TQM, senior management has allotted nearly $100,000 during 1990 in support of PAT recommendations, including $17,000 for a computer installation and $25,000 for the purchase of facsimile machines to improve communication between wards and the pharmacy.

PATs that address cross-functional issues are chartered or "blessed" by the Quality Council and have specific "process owners." Owners of cross-functional PATs are typically members of executive management. Teams that deal with smaller issues (that is, within one department) are encouraged to form without the Council's approval; staff refer to these teams as "bootleg" PATs. The chartering process allows the Quality Council to provide support to and keep up-to-date on a PAT's activities. As part of the chartering process, each new PAT receives some initial training to help in its formation and initiation. The team's first two meetings are spent in training—learning team

---

Table 2.1. A Sample of WPMC's PAT Activities (continued)

the order to transfer and ends when notification is complete. The improvement should reduce errors and rework and save resources.

Lab PAT. Reduce turnaround time for STAT lab requests from the emergency room and intensive care unit. Reduce to less than one hour from the time STAT is ordered to the time it is delivered to the emergency room or the intensive care unit for 80% of requests.

"Megawhopper" PAT. Investigates a patient's course of care for the breast evaluation process from the time a mammography is ordered until surgery. Improve patient care. (See page 64 for more on this PAT.)

X-ray/Surgery PAT. Reduce delivery time of exposed film to the operating room for use in surgical procedures.

Same-Day Surgery PAT. Improve process from physician's decision to schedule for same day surgery to the point of the patient's arrival for surgery. Should reduce excess paperwork in the record, increase completion of required patient trips to the medical center for same-day surgery workup, and decrease unnecessary preoperative tests.

Lab PAT. Improve process of obtaining complete lab slips so that all necessary demographic data is on the form. Begins when the provider orders a lab and ends with lab results being posted to the computer. Improving the process should result in a dramatic reduction in incomplete lab slips from the current 70%, reduce repeat labs, and reduce staff and patient frustration.

Source: *Developed by Terence T. Cunningham, Colonel, USAF, MSC, Administrator, USAF Medical Center, Wright-Patterson, Dayton, Ohio, 1991. Reprinted with permission.*

skills, TQM tools, meeting management techniques, and the FOCUS-PDCA process improvement approach, which WPMC adopted from Quorum (see pages 34–35). If PATs need further assistance, they can turn to their PAT support group, which is made up of three to five people of whom at least one is a Quality Council member. The process owner, PAT leader, and facilitator meet regularly with the support group. (Although the process owners are members of executive management, they are not members of the support group that guides their own PATs.) The support group mentors and monitors the PAT and updates the Quality Council on their activities. Essentially, the support group is the interface between the PATs and the Quality Council.

The use of storyboards and storybooks has also assisted teams in getting underway and communicating their activities. Storyboards display the team's activities according to the steps in the FOCUS-PDCA cycle. More involved than the boards, storybooks walk team leaders through all the steps involved in team formation and provide a medium to record the team's activities.

A case study (page 57) tells the story of the inpatient medication management PAT and how the use of an ingenious data-collection tool, the Proctor's Patented Pucky Collector, helped team members arrive at a creative solution to the defective inpatient medication management process.

QA/QI Relationship

QA is not integrated with TQM at WPMC. Although staff are using TQM concepts and tools to improve QA, it is a separate function. Staff do not feel TQM can evolve from QA since QA is considered to be only a part of TQM. TQM is viewed as a total management system, which is philosophically different and broader in scope than QA. A key reason management is hesitant to connect the two is the bad reputation QA has had at WPMC. Having little computerized support, clinical staff often had to collect data manually, which became very burdensome. In addition, QA did not focus on processes so QA activities rarely led to an improvement. Staff began to see QA as a "non–value-added" activity done to satisfy the Joint Commission and military regulations.

In its effort to make the transition from QA to TQM, the medical center has adopted a patient-focused quality improvement program, which is a collaborative model of patient care assessment. Care

(continued on page 64)

Case Study
The Story of WPMC's Inpatient Medication Management PAT

Opportunity for improvement

The medical staff were concerned. They expected their patients to be medicated according to orders. The medication nurses were frustrated and angry. They were concerned that pharmacy personnel were incompetent and uncaring. Passing medications with the unit dose system was a game of roulette—the medication was there two thirds of the time, but one third of the time it was missing, wrong, or in an inappropriate strength.

Meanwhile, the pharmacy staff were trying hard to make the unit dose system work and were tired of being blamed for the problem; they felt they were victims of problems over which they had no control. With no automated delivery system, both nursing and pharmacy personnel were jointly responsible for hand carrying all copies of physician's orders to the pharmacy for medication dispensing. To make matters worse, the copies were often unreadable. The pharmacy staff felt the nurses were too quick to point the finger. The hostility level was high, resulting in frequent confrontations between nursing and pharmacy personnel.

Poor quality pharmacy service was being driven by poor communication, outdated internal pharmacy procedures, and long-standing medical center delivery problems. As a result, morale was rock-bottom in both departments as nursing and pharmacy supervisors attempted to manage each daily crisis. The problem with inpatient medication management was even more surprising when one considers that Wright-Patterson Medical Center (WPMC) was reopened in 1989 as the most modern of all Air Force hospitals. No expense was spared to provide space, staff, skills, and training.

Process Improvement Method

The inpatient medication management PAT (IMM/PAT) was chartered by WPMC's Quality Council in May 1990 and began meeting weekly. Using the FOCUS-PDCA process improvement approach explained on pages 34–35, the team began investigating the problem.

Find the problem. The team's mandate was ambitious—"fix the broken inpatient medication management system." Before teams at WPMC begin, the Quality Council, along with the process owner, team leader, and facilitator, create an initial "opportunity statement" that defines where the team will begin and end its process evaluation. When trying to "focus on the problem," the IMM/PAT learned its opportunity statement was too broad. Fortunately, it eventually narrowed the scope to more manageable boundaries.

The team's final opportunity statement was narrowed to "An important opportunity exists with the process of communication, filling and delivering unit dose medication orders between the medical/surgical wards and inpatient pharmacy, beginning with the nurse taking off the order for the medication and ending with delivery of the medication to the nursing unit. The current process results in a large number of medication discrepancies which cause great mental anguish and hostility. Improvements should result in reduced discrepancies, reduced rework, improved relationships, and a better working environment."

Organize a team. Although the team was organized around personnel directly involved in the medication distribution process, the team leader was a psychiatrist and an occupational therapist was named facilitator. Other team members, including charge nurses, pharmacists, unit clerks, and the hospital attorney, were

- Major Brian Proctor, MD, staff psychiatrist, team leader;
- Major Bill Wells, medical legal consultant;
- Major Carol Pierce, charge nurse;
- Major Patty Hirshouer, charge nurse;
- Captain John D. James, chief, inpatient pharmacy services;
- Captain Laura Murphy, discharge planning nurse;
- Captain Carl Richie, supervisor, inpatient pharmacy;
- First Lieutenant Mary Bedard, supervisor, pharmacy admixture service;
- First Lieutenant Sandra Moore, occupational therapist, team facilitator;
- Master Sergeant Al Kostrab, technician supervisor, inpatient pharmacy;
- Charlene Black, unit secretary; and
- Bettie Melton, unit secretary.

Clarify the process. The team first plotted on a flowchart the medication management process to identify internal customers and "problem" steps. When completed, the flowchart wrapped around three walls of the meeting room. The flowchart started with the physician writing the medication order and ended with medication delivery to the nursing unit. Next, the team had to identify primary problems and key quality characteristics. Members had to substitute objective and measurable facts in place of subjective opinions to identify the true problem. According to the Pareto principle, 80% of a problem is caused by 20% of its elements. Nursing problems identified were missing medications, wrong medications, and correct medication but wrong strength. Pharmacy problems included having to call the ward to clarify an illegible order, being called by the ward when the nurse could not find a medication but had sent an order, and receiving a call from the nurse for a missing medication when pharmacy could not find an order. Figure 2.A (below) provides a draft of the Ishikawa or cause-and-effect diagram. The team collected baseline data for these various problem elements, both on the nursing unit and in the pharmacy department, in an effort to sort out the "significant few" elements from the "trivial many."

The team leader devised an ingenious solution to the usual historical difficulties of attaining accurate data when people are asked to fill out forms—the "Proctor's Patent Pucky Collector" (PPPC). The PPPC is a shoe box with four empty Pringles™ Potato Chip cans glued to the bottom against one side and a supply of marbles (see Figure 2.B, page 60). Each can is labeled with a specific problem element. The four cans were labeled "missing med," "wrong med," "wrong strength," and "other." To collect data on nursing units, the nurse placed the PPPC on the medication cart he or she pushed about a unit. When the nurse discovered, for example, that a needed medication was not in the drawer, a marble was dropped in the can labeled "missing med." The PPPC was used in the pharmacy in the same manner. Data were gathered over a one-week period in July 1990. Each type of discrepancy was tallied separately and calculated as a percentage of the total. These

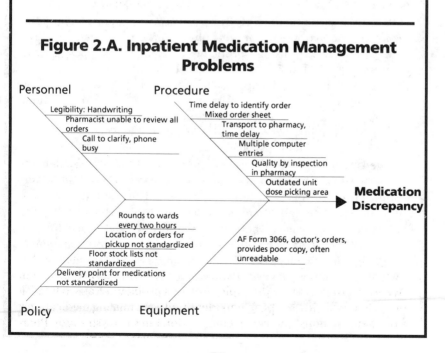

Figure 2.A. Inpatient Medication Management Problems

Personnel

Procedure

Legibility: Handwriting
Pharmacist unable to review all orders
Call to clarify, phone busy

Time delay to identify order
Mixed order sheet
Transport to pharmacy, time delay
Multiple computer entries
Quality by inspection in pharmacy
Outdated unit dose picking area

▶ **Medication Discrepancy**

Rounds to wards every two hours
Location of orders for pickup not standardized
Floor stock lists not standardized
Delivery point for medications not standardized

AF Form 3066, doctor's orders, provides poor copy, often unreadable

Policy

Equipment

Figure 2.B. Procter's Patent Pucky Collector

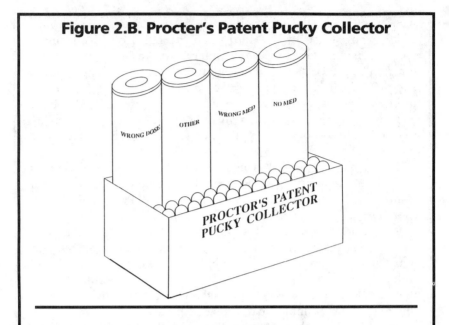

values were used to identify key problems and later served as control comparisons.

Understand the process variance. Interpreting the flowchart and the PPPC data helped the team understand process variance. The flowchart described a very complex process and identified multiple internal customers. Nearly one-third of all steps involved handling or transporting a carbonless copy of the original physician's order. When the PPPC data were analyzed, distinct problems were identified. (The Pareto diagrams provided in Figure 2.C, page 61, illustrate these data.) The primary problem for nursing was clearly missing medications. Of 51 total events counted, 43 were missing medications (84%), despite a pharmacist matching the pharmacy medication profile against the nursing medication cardex (100% inspections) for accuracy every day. In the pharmacy, calling to clarify an order represented 63% of events counted (39 of 60 total). Several key issues were identified: handling the physician's order required multiple non–value-added steps and was a significant source of variance in the process. The resulting copy was poor and often illegible, and, since all copies of orders were hand-carried to the pharmacy, there was a significant time delay from the time the order was written until it was received by pharmacy personnel. The key quality characteristic for the nursing service customer was the correct medication delivered and available in a timely manner. The key quality characteristic for the pharmacy customer was a legible copy of the physician's medication order delivered and available in a timely manner.

Select an improvement. Based on their findings, the team's suggested improvement was to use facsimile transmission machines (fax) to transmit a copy of the original physician's order to the pharmacy.

Plan–Do–Check–Act. The team planned a fax machine trial to see if both nursing and pharmacy's key quality characteristics could be improved. The IMM/PAT planned a fax machine trial on two nursing units. Since Ward 3 West was the site of all previous data collection, it served as the test site. Ward 4 West, a smaller unit, refined the fax procedure prior to starting the trial on 3 West. Three area office equipment companies loaned fax machines for evaluation and trained personnel in their operation. After the fax procedure was refined, the PPPC was used to count medication discrepancies, which decreased by 46%. The second week, total discrepancies decreased by 65%. The bar graph depicted in Figure 2.D (page 62) illustrates this significant reduction in discrepancies. During this time, the pharmacy department did not reconcile the nursing unit medex to the pharmacy profile.

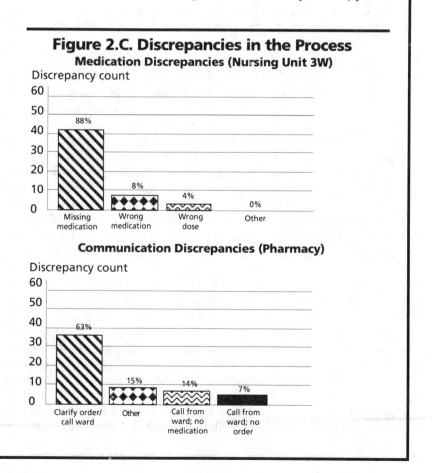

Figure 2.C. Discrepancies in the Process
Medication Discrepancies (Nursing Unit 3W)

Discrepancy count

Missing medication	Wrong medication	Wrong dose	Other
88%	8%	4%	0%

Communication Discrepancies (Pharmacy)

Discrepancy count

Clarify order/ call ward	Other	Call from ward; no medication	Call from ward; no order
63%	15%	14%	7%

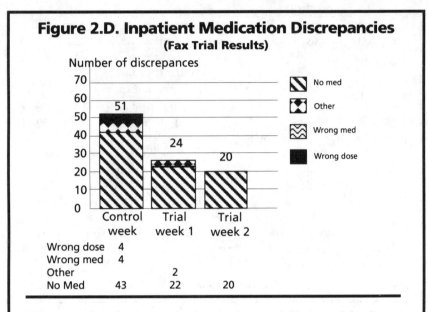

Figure 2.D. Inpatient Medication Discrepancies
(Fax Trial Results)

Number of discrepances

No med	Other	Wrong med

Legend:
- No med
- Other
- Wrong med
- Wrong dose

	Control week	Trial week 1	Trial week 2
	51	24	20
Wrong dose	4		
Wrong med	4		
Other		2	
No Med	43	22	20

This stopped expensive, useless inspections and eliminated the discrepancies rather than correcting them when they occurred.

The final step in the PDCA cycle is to *act*, is to hold the gain. The IMM/PAT recommended to the Quality Council that fax machines be purchased and placed on all nursing units and in the pharmacy and then further recommended examining fax machines for use in addressing communication problems with other ancillary services. The pharmacy continues to collect and monitor data.

The PDCA cycle's importance to quality improvement cannot be overemphasized. By testing the suggested improvement, its utility is proved and it is implemented, or it is disproved and the team starts over. If the suggestion is implemented, the team should test the process again at some predetermined point in the future to assure the improvement is permanent and the process does not in fact "lose ground."

Summary

As of August 1991, the fax network installation is being completed. The total integration of fax machines into the medical center was delayed while WPMC was called to directly support activities during Operation Desert Storm. Still, the team has documented significant quality improvement since June 1990. Medical discrepancies were 93 per nursing unit per week. Currently on those units where the faxes are in place, medication discrepancies for the entire unit dose system within the medical center have decreased, and turnaround time for medication orders is now less than two hours. Most important, the quality of inpatient pharmacy service as defined by the nursing service customer is enormously improved.

Although rare, missing meds still occur—they are usually the result of variance in the new system. A missing medication request form was designed to allow the nurse to fax a request for a missing medication. Pharmacy sends the needed medication on receipt of the form. Data collected from the forms are used to track the missing med rate for the entire medical center on a run chart by day, week, and month. As the team continues to gather and track these data (see Figure 2.E, below), they are better able to understand the variance within this system and better equipped to continually improve the quality of service.

Other benefits include improved professional relationships among physicians, nurses, and pharmacists and real cost avoidance from improved efficiency and reduction of waste and rework. Physicians are pleased with the promptness and accuracy of the new medication distribution process. Medication nurses are confident that all medications the patients need are available when they need them. Nurses no longer waste valuable patient care time looking for medications. Pharmacy personnel enjoy the atmosphere of respect and support as they provide a quality service to nursing. Significant time savings are realized through improved efficiency. The team estimates that both nursing and pharmacy combined have saved one or two full-time personnel. Staff no longer have to look for meds or hand-carry medication orders between nursing unit and pharmacy. The team subsequently discovered substantial cost avoidance when a study of returned intravenous admixtures indicated return rates were reduced from between 25% to 100% after implementation of the fax machines.

Source: This case study was written and developed by Captain John D. James, USAF, BSC (PharmD, MBA) Chief, Inpatient Pharmacy Services, USAF Medical Center Wright-Patterson/SGHP, Wright-Patterson Air Force Base, OH 45433-5300. Captain James will gladly answer questions submitted by letter on any aspect of this case. Correspondence should include a phone number. Time and work load prohibit taking questions directly over the phone.

Figure 2.E. Missing Unit Dose Meds
May 1991—All Wards

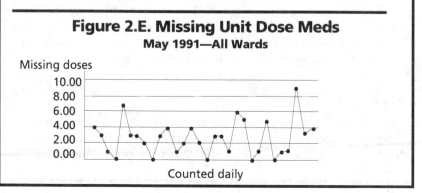

(continued from page 56)

throughout the organization is beginning to be perceived as the result of a team effort, and accountability is seen as the team's responsibility, not only the physician's. While the Joint Commission medical staff standards (that is, medical record review, surgical case review) are strictly adhered to, nurses now join in the review to determine quality of nursing care issues. Physician privileges and credentialing processes have not been altered.

WPMC is also trying to "weed out" monitoring those indicators "that are non-value added," Foster said. While they are still monitoring key indicators such as mortality, morbidity, and nosocomial infections and completing quarterly reports, D'Aquila-Lloyd and her staff have worked with departments across the hospital to drastically reduce the amount of monitoring done. Areas that have historically been monitored by traditional QA tools are being assessed within clinical process improvement teams. These are multidisciplinary team efforts that involve the assessment and improvement of processes that are related to one or more of the following:

- Optimization of a process or outcome of care;
- Improvement of resource utilization;
- Enhancement of patient satisfaction; and
- Minimization of the risk of danger or illness associated with care.

FOCUS-PDCA is the method by which clinical processes are evaluated. The approach is focused on processes rather than individual practitioners. Staff believe these areas would be better improved when explored as processes rather than monitored as outcomes. For example, previously the ten-step monitoring and evaluation process was performed to evaluate the 1,200 indicators on the nursing units at WPMC; now this list of 1,200 has been whittled down to about 20 for the entire medical center. Data are collected for these few indicators and, if problems are identified, collaborative teams are developed to identify the source or cause. In WPMC's experience to date, each problem identified was a process problem, not a provider problem.

The "population at risk for breast disease" PAT, nicknamed the "megawhopper process" PAT because it is such a complex process, helped staff understand the switch in emphasis from QA to QI. The PAT was formed after customers complained they were not getting notified of mammography results in a timely fashion. There was too much time between diagnosis and surgery. Investigating the complaints, D'Aquila-Lloyd's staff charted the major events of 29 cases; tremendous variation among cases was revealed. Representatives from seven areas—administration, oncology, nursing, radiology, surgery, gynecology, and primary care—formed the PAT, which devised a comprehensive macrolevel flowchart of a patient's course through the breast liaison process, from the time a mammography was ordered until surgery. The resulting huge flowchart caused a paradigm shift throughout the organization. The flowchart

- convinced staff how important focusing on processes is;
- softened the barriers between departments;
- helped convince staff of the importance of moving toward TQM;
- promoted awareness of the need for developing a more collaborative culture; and
- became the stimulus for further research to look at other major processes that occur within the medical center that can be improved to the benefit of their ultimate customer.

Education

When WPMC began their TQM efforts, staff were trained on a volunteer basis. However, it soon became apparent that this method did not provide the broad base of senior and junior personnel needed to support the rollout of TQM. A major disadvantage within a military hospital moving to TQM is the forced turnover of staff, including the commander, every three to four years. WPMC has approached this barrier from several angles.

The Quality Council has begun an aggressive campaign to educate a critical mass of staff that will withstand the 20.4% annual turnover. They are cascading TQM through the organization by training one department at a time. The Quality Council's goal is to have 1,200 supervisors and 600 nonsupervisory employees trained in TQM by the end of fiscal year 1991. Unfortunately, the hospital is limited by the number of training slots the base can provide. Through an agreement with AFIT, medical center staff are allowed to attend a course in TQM methods and statistical process control that augments base education courses. Working with a budget of $50,000 for fiscal year 1991, the QI coach and executive staff at WPMC have developed other curricula to supplement the base and AFIT courses, including a three-day TQM course based on HCA's Q-101 course. WPMC's course uses examples specific to WPMC and is taught by members of the Quality Council.

Other in-house education courses being developed include basic statistical process control, advanced statistical process control, and a jump-start course for PATs. Members of the Quality Council as well as other key management staff teach these in-house courses.

To reach newcomers, senior management used an existing sponsorship program to help orient new employees about TQM before they arrive at the medical center. Approximately one to three months before new employees start they receive a letter that explains the TQM initiative at WPMC. They are asked to read an attached article and encouraged to read Mary Walton's *The Deming Management Method* before beginning work. The QI coach also provides newcomers with a 60-minute briefing on TQM as part of orientation.

The hospital identified the development of facilitators and trainers as a top priority early on. A facilitator training course is also being developed. The Quality Council carefully selects teachers from the medical center staff to become instructors and facilitators for PATs.

There are many other less formal methods for learning about TQM concepts at WPMC. The Upton Society, the book club established by Roadman for senior management, has become an open forum for all levels of the organization to discuss current TQM topics once a month. The TQM office also maintains a large selection of books and videos on management issues that are available to staff.

QI Supports

Tied closely to the success of WPMC's TQM strategy is the resolution of many practical issues, such as the provision of process-oriented data to teams, recognition of team activities, and a mechanism to receive ongoing customer feedback.

Customer-supplier feedback. WPMC's early emphasis on the customer led Roadman to charter the feedback loop PAT in July 1989 specifically to examine the methods being used to gather feedback from customers, particularly patients. The PAT developed a flowchart of the ideal process for patient feedback (see Figure 2.2, page 67) and has arrived at several methods to increase access to patient opinion. A survey of patients and staff revealed that the existing method for surveying inpatients and outpatients was ineffective. The return rate was low, and there was no centralized control over the surveys sent out. Many departments sent out their own surveys, and the results were difficult to track and report to the executive staff. The PAT developed a standardized survey for inpatients and outpatients and got permis-

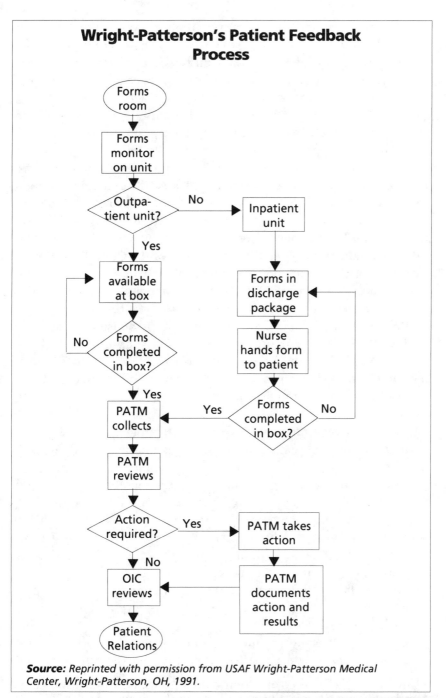

Wright-Patterson's Patient Feedback Process

Source: *Reprinted with permission from USAF Wright-Patterson Medical Center, Wright-Patterson, OH, 1991.*

Figure 2.2. Wright-Patterson's feedback loop PAT developed a flowchart of the ideal process for patient feedback.

sion to purchase an optical scanner that easily compiles the data gathered. Cindy Huffman, patient relations coordinator, provides trend analysis of the survey data and patient complaints to the executive committee and each department. She uses control charts to display the data. Departments are still encouraged to conduct their own surveys, but "they have to be value-added" (for example, to further investigate an issue revealed by the organizationwide survey), Huffman said.

Information systems. WPMC presently has a patchwork of automated medical systems and software that includes 21 different mini computers and 465 personal computers. The 15-member management information systems (MIS) department is currently able to provide information to PATs or design systems to track data as needed. However, staff are looking forward to the installation of the Composite Health Care System, which is a single patient data base being developed by the Department of Defense. The front-end system will support order entry, result reporting, administration, QA, and resource management. Providers will be able to enter data at the bedside.

The MIS department provides additional support to the TQM effort at WPMC by serving as consultants to PATs and helping members determine what types of information they may need. MIS is developing a course on statistical process control that they will offer to interested staff.

Reward and recognition. WPMC is investigating how to shift the military's traditional reward system, which primarily rewards an individual for personal performance (for example, with medals), to promote the contributions individuals make as members of teams. Job descriptions of military personnel have been revised to include references to quality improvement activities, and an award, "The Quality Coin," was established to honor staff for their work on teams. Unfortunately, although an outstanding honor, the criteria for the Quality Coin are "so stringent we can not award very many," according to B. Murray. Applicants must demonstrate knowledge of customers, processes, and statistics. The Quality Council is investigating a more immediate reward structure.

Celebrations are another method to recognize the work of teams. The hospital recently had its first TQM Sharing Day where several PATs presented their stories in the hospital auditorium. Other PATs set up their storyboards in the hallway, and staff were given maps to direct them to each storyboard. To demonstrate the importance of this event, Anderson informed the medical center that it was understood if staff had to schedule their departments at half staff on that day.

Benchmarking. The Quality Council is actively engaged in benchmarking with other TQM organizations. They visit other hospitals and companies implementing TQM.

Physician Involvement

An advantage unique to a military hospital is that "physicians come with the package," Cunningham said. Because physicians are employed solely by the medical center, WPMC has not had difficulty engaging physicians in TQM. Taking advantage of a captive audience, WPMC engaged the medical staff from the very beginning. Most PATs include physicians and, as heads of medical departments, physicians are driving the rollout of TQM throughout the organization. The relatively simple engagement of physicians in TQM has led staff to conclude that the problem between physicians and TQM boils down to a very practical issue—time. Unlike the private sector, physicians at WPMC do not have to see patients to ensure their incomes and so they are more willing to take the time to learn about TQM.

Leaders at WPMC have found the following methods helpful in developing physicians' enthusiasm for TQM:

- Emphasizing that TQM looks at processes rather than individuals;
- Identifying physicians considered leaders within the hospital who would lead the rollout of TQM among the medical staff;
- Emphasizing that TQM problem solving is a form of the scientific method;
- Illustrating how physicians are suppliers as well as customers (for example, demonstrate through a flowchart how an illegibly signed record creates rework);
- Demonstrating that TQM is a value-added activity, as opposed to the way they had practiced QA; and
- Discovering a method to break through the language barrier that TQM produces (that is, TQM words sound like a foreign language to many physicians).

Conclusion

Rather than being hampered by the traditionally stringent rules and regulations of a military facility, staff are stimulated within the culture at WPMC. As shown throughout this chapter, staff are creatively seeking innovative ways to color outside the lines. TQM tools and the problem-solving process have provided staff with the methods they need to be empowered. Although staff have run into some unique barriers to implementing TQM within a military hospital (for example, the forced turnover of personnel), many of the lessons staff have learned are applicable to any type of hospital making the transition to TQM.

3 Lowering the Water Line

Memorial Hospital and Health System South Bend, Indiana

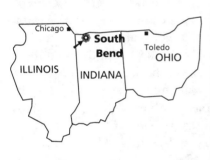

Type of hospital: Not-for-profit community
Scope of services: General medical and surgical
Beds: 463, with average census of 311
Extent of TQM involvement: After a commitment in 1988, Memorial has made headway along two tracks—systems and departments. Eighty percent of departments now have their own quality plans, and senior management and the board are putting the finishing touches on an organizationwide strategic plan that includes visionary goals and tactics to meet them.

Special aspects of Memorial's TQM activities:
— Composite TQM approach based on Juran
— Antecedent environment that emphasizes customer relations and empowerment
— Move to shared governance
— Rollout of TQM along two tracks
— Value-based planning process involving visioning
— Model to determine cost of quality
— Program to reward managers based in part on customer feedback
— Development of benchmarking

Empowerment is more than a buzzword at Memorial Hospital and Health System; it is a responsibility. Every staff member contributes to his or her department's vision and quality plan, nursing units are operated by shared or self-governance agreements, and each department manager's salary is tied to quality. When describing the culture at Memorial, Philip A. Newbold, chief executive officer and president, compares Memorial to a ship: the lower the waterline, the more room for risk taking and innovation. Newbold stresses that if changes are made below the waterline without the knowledge of how different functions within Memorial affect each other, those changes could end up drilling holes in the supporting structure of the organization.[1] Believing the largest breakthroughs can often occur through "skunk work," or unsanctioned entrepreneurship, Newbold keeps the waterline low at Memorial and encourages staff to creatively improve those functions and processes above the waterline.

Nancy Jelsma, quality clinical specialist, said there was "a certain energy at Memorial" even before the arrival of Newbold and total quality management (TQM). Staff had been taking empowerment courses and were "encouraged to be creative and take power . . . on a day-to-day level." But the wall-sized plaque bearing the word "Excellence" that was hung in Memorial's lobby eight years ago rang hollow until TQM was introduced. "TQM was the spark ... it supported the energy," Jelsma said. The difference was the management commitment and the structure (for example, problem-solving approach, tools, department quality plans) that came with TQM. Linda Betz, director of nursing management systems, describes TQM as "more of a philosophical integration." Now she says the "quality emphasis is the administrative emphasis. We hear as much now about customer needs as about the budget," Betz said. While staff throughout Memorial are busily investigating ways to cut rework and improve processes using TQM techniques, Newbold and his senior management maintain an acute awareness of skunk work that might strike below the waterline. Through the two-track rollout that Memorial has adopted—a systems improvement track and a department quality planning track—Memorial is creating an environment that encourages innovation down through the line level but ensures that top management directs improvement in those macro level processes that fall below the water line. So while staff create flowcharts and cause-and-effect diagrams to investigate those processes close to them, senior management monitors and designs organizationwide systems.

Description and Demographics

Staff at Memorial share the same spirit as the fighting Irish down the street. About two hours east of Chicago, South Bend is famous as a university town, housing the University of Notre Dame and other colleges. Memorial and Notre Dame are two of the largest employers in St Joseph County, which is Memorial's primary service area with a population of 250,000. The largest medical center (463 beds) in northern Indiana, Memorial receives patients from an 11-county area around St Joseph County. Thirty-three percent of Memorial's patient days represent Medicare and Medicaid patients. Besides medical/surgical services, patients are also attracted to Memorial for its cancer center, rehabilitation institute, regional center for mother and child, heart institute, emergency and trauma center, and behavioral health service. The organization shares many of its 350 medical staff members with St Joseph's Medical Center in South Bend, its largest competitor.

Memorial Hospital is part of a larger corporation, Memorial Health System, that manages a broad spectrum of health-related services throughout the community, including immediate care centers, family practice centers, home care division, pharmaceutical services, medical supply, and occupational health services and assistance to local employers, including worker's compensation, treatment and assessment, and physical examinations.

History

Newbold arrived at Memorial in the fall of 1987 looking for a way to go beyond traditional customer service methods. He felt Memorial needed "something up front to avoid and minimize the errors." "Frank's Place Group" was created; Newbold named the group after the local tavern where he and select senior management met each week to discuss the direction of the organization. Eventually, it became apparent that the Frank's Place Group needed to expand. Soon thereafter a weekend retreat was scheduled, and over 50 managers and other staff attended. Newbold realized over the two days that his "staff had the necessary energy and discipline" to pursue a more comprehensive quality effort. He went back to his notes from a Tom Peter's course and saw those ideas as a new way to manage. Newbold decided to launch a quality revolution at Memorial.

A team of senior managers began to further research TQM concepts and study the different approaches, such as those of Deming and Juran. An important part of the team's research was benchmarking with other TQM organizations. The team, plus several board members, visited Florida Power & Light in Miami; Alliant Health Systems in Louisville, Kentucky; Rush-Presbyterian-St Luke's Medical Center in Chicago; and others to carefully study how the methods of these organizations might be applied at Memorial.

In May 1989, administrative staff gathered to begin applying the team's research directly to Memorial. In what Doug Mosel, director of quality and organization development, described as a "hard-working two days," administrative staff set about defining what quality meant for Memorial and what qualities the organization valued. The process was "a way of connecting to our organizational history," Mosel said. Reviewing the different approaches, senior management decided to develop their own hybrid approach to TQM that leans toward Juran and strongly emphasizes strategic planning (see "Philosophy"). Newbold stresses that going with a hybrid approach over a turnkey approach was an important decision point. "Although . . . a consultant would probably never have allowed us to end up in some of the cul-de-sacs we have found ourselves in," Newbold said, "I think we ended up with a better product." In another symbolic move, senior management named their TQM effort "Quality Through People" and developed a logo that emphasized that "it was staff who were going to turn Memorial into a quality organization," Mosel said.

Once the philosophical structure for its TQM effort was in place, management began rolling it out. The focus in the initial years has primarily been on devising a structure and strategy to support their effort. Management established a Quality Council to oversee the roll-out and dedicated staff to provide support. The Quality Council is chaired by Newbold and includes the same senior management that are on Memorial's administrative council. They meet twice a month for at least two hours to discuss TQM-related issues. The responsibilities of the Quality Council include planning and oversight of Memorial's two-track approach. The Council charters quality improvement teams (QITs) and develops organizationwide strategy. The quality and organization development staff, directed by Mosel, supports both tracks. The department provides training, coaching, and facilitating. Mosel is assisted by Jelsma, who primarily supports the rollout of TQM in the clinical areas. The board also was involved in the effort from the beginning and is heavily involved in devising the strategic plan, with its strong emphasis on quality.

Believing strongly that TQM must be leader driven, Memorial has concentrated on educating top and middle managers in TQM concepts and tools (see "Education"). Pilot teams were formed to test the concepts staff had learned, and the department planning method was tested in several departments. All departments are now developing their own quality plans. Midway into 1991, senior management and the board are devising a long-term strategy that provides an organizationwide focus to their endeavors. This, combined with department-level activities, puts Memorial well on its way toward 1995, which they have identified as the year of "real system results and performance."

Philosophy

Staff at Memorial have taken methods and ideas from a variety of sources and woven them into a package that is uniquely their own and fits the culture at Memorial. They devised their own seven-step problem-solving approach that combines Juran and Deming features, chose awareness materials from Organizational Dynamics, Inc in Burlington, Massachusetts, developed facilitator and TQM team training based on Juran, studied critical pathways through site visits and a National Demonstration Project workshop, and recently concluded an intensive visioning process based on Senge.[2] Senior management defined quality as "exceeding customer expectations by doing right things right." A pyramid (see Figure 3.1, page 76) was devised to illustrate the principles the Quality Council found key to TQM, and the organizational values—quality, respect, efficiency, and innovation—were placed at the bottom of the pyramid to illustrate their importance. Although homegrown, Memorial's TQM approach is largely indebted to Juran. Core to Memorial's philosophy is understanding Juran's trilogy—quality planning, quality assurance (QA), and quality improvement (QI).[3]

Memorial's two-track approach is the organization's route to becoming an entirely new organization. The systems track, which focuses on cross-departmental opportunities for improvement, and the department quality planning track run along parallel lines. While both senior management and department managers are involved in quality planning, QA, and QI, the Quality Council and the board are developing organizationwide objectives and goals and assessing macro processes and functions (also referred to as "systems"). Department managers and their staffs are more concerned with department-

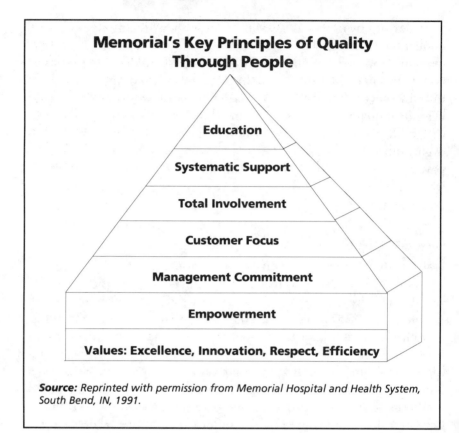

Figure 3.1. This pyramid emphasizes the importance that management at Memorial places on its organizational values. These values essentially support the TQM effort at Memorial.

specific goals and micro processes that affect them directly. According to Newbold, an organization will "get the greatest leverage by improving the macro level" processes and redesigning systems. In their initial enthusiasm, QI teams were "mapping detailed flowcharts," Mosel said. While this step was probably useful in initial training, Mosel emphasizes that systems-oriented teams "should instead look at high-level flowcharts and look at details only when they need to focus."

Rolling out TQM along the two tracks is one approach Memorial is using to resolve the conflict between what is above and below the water line. Newbold acknowledges that innovation often comes through skunk work, but he is also concerned about the effect a "skunk" improvement could have on a core system, such as medical records or admitting. Within "some core systems, staff don't know the impact" of a proposed change down the line, Newbold said. "That's where we need management people involved." He suggests keeping skunk woɪ at the micro level and assigning macro level planning to senior management. "It's okay to experiment with late trays or change things about turnaround times . . . [we] need lots of experimentation" in these areas. Training will also control harmful skunk work. As staff begin to understand systems theory, they are becoming less likely to jump to hasty solutions. Another approach Memorial is using to align skunk work is through an intensive process of "visioning," which is explained further in the next section.

Strategy

In line with the organization's emphasis on planning, Memorial began developing a systemwide three-year strategic plan in the fall of 1990. In what staff termed "value-based planning," management and board members began by projecting what they wanted Memorial to be like in the year 2000. Value-based planning begins by defining the organization's vision, which in turn springs from the hospital's values. This approach differs from traditional strategic planning, which often springs from environmental and budgetary constraints. Memorial began by asking "What can we be?" and "What do we want?" rather than "How can we meet budget?" While Memorial cannot ignore financial, regulatory, and other worries, senior management is refusing to be limited by those constraints up-front. Instead they began with a vision and are developing a long-term strategy for how that vision can be pursued. As annual tactics are devised to meet their strategic goals, financial, facility, budgetary, and quality responsibilities will gradually be "integrated" so that ultimately vision and quality drive the overall process. Table 3.1 (page 78) illustrates the contrast between traditional and value-based planning.

Management brought the results of the new planning approach to a two-day board forum in May 1991 that included senior managers, board members, and medical staff leaders. From the work of earlier "visioning" sessions with over 300 people, the forum endorsed five major themes for Memorial to pursue between or in the year 2000:

- *Quality:* Exceeding customer expectations and professional standards by doing right things right;

- *Enhancing community health:* Strengthening the relationship between Memorial and the community;

- *Medical staff leadership:* Continued development, vitality, and leadership of the medical staff of Memorial;

Table 3.1. Differences Between Memorial's Value-Based Planning and Traditional Planning

Traditional Planning	Value-Based Planning
Begins with environmental reconnaissance where strategic options are developed based on both internal and external constraints	Begins outside the realm of constraints and ask "What can we be? What do we want?" Value-based planning begins by defining the vision
Often conducted in isolation from other planning processes	Integrates strategic, capital, facilities, and quality plans
Completes a document and is concluded	Implements specific actions to move from current reality toward the vision
Derived from logic (that is, an extension of the "present state")	Rooted in shared values and a common vision
Forms strategic options within environmental constraints	Reaches beyond perceived constraints to define what is possible
Extends *history* into the future and seeks to optimize the *probable*	Extends *values* into the future to identify the *possible*. "Visioning" is the first step in choosing and creating a preferred future, not as a tactical extension of the past
	Enhances traditional planning; it does not eliminate it. Starts by creating a vision of what future is preferred, designs a strategy for how the vision can be pursued, and then builds an operational plan to link budgets with annual tactical activities

Source: Adapted from materials developed by Memorial Hospital and Health System, South Bend, Indiana. Reprinted with permission.

- *Regionalization/technology:* Providing health care services to serve the regional community; and

- *Education:* Providing a linkage with the community to encourage a positive environment focused on the education of employees and the community about health care.

Asked to prioritize these objectives, the board decided to concentrate on two: enhancing community health and improving regionalization/ technology. Teams composed of senior management, board members, physicians, and staff were assigned to investigate and plan the rollout in each of these areas. The board then identified seven services within the organization where staff should begin addressing the two objectives: non–hospital services, hospital outpatient services, cardiology, oncology, rehabilitation, mother/child, and medical/surgical. Other teams, composed of a similar mix of people, were charged with assessing the current environment and devising an action plan to enhance community health and improve regionalization/technology within each service area—a process termed "integration." Part of this integration process was the inclusion of budgetary and other constraints. For example, the team devising strategy within cardiology went through the following steps:

- Analyzing the environment within cardiology, both internally (for example, the medical staff, finances) and externally (for example, industry and customer trends, payer mix);

- Determining strengths, weaknesses, opportunities, and threats (SWOTs analysis) within cardiology;

- Identifying opportunities that would support collaboration and outreach within cardiology;

- Selecting a strategy appropriate to integration of requirements (for example, financial targets, facilities plan, quality targets);

- Identifying three-year goals, which included quality indicators for utilization, margins, capital, quality, community health status indicator(s), and regional network indicator(s); and

- Devising a one-year action plan that included programs, access, pricing, promotion, budget, and quality.

Action plans for achieving enhanced community health and regionalization/technology in each of the seven hospital services will be implemented by January 1992. At the end of 1992, initial results on the success of the measures taken in each area, including indicator rates, will be provided.

Some departments and divisions are preparing their own visions for the future. While a department's vision may be slightly different from the organizationwide vision, members of senior management continually stress the importance of departmental visions "heading in the same general direction" as the organization's vision, said George Soper, senior vice-president and chief operating officer. The diagrams below illustrate how a department's vision can be unique but still relate to the entire organization's vision. Senior managers have held visioning sessions with some staff that explain the importance of a shared organizational vision, and many staff, particularly nurses and physicians, have been involved in developing the vision of Memorial in the year 2000. As one staff member said, "empowerment without a shared vision is counterproductive."

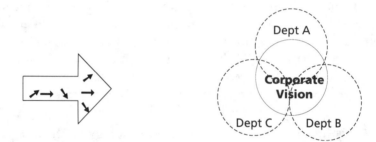

Each department and/or unit at Memorial develops its own annual department quality plan. As part of this planning process, department managers work with their staff to identify their customers' requirements, define indicators to assess how well they are meeting customer needs, and develop action plans to improve their process. Table 3.2 (page 81) provides the steps involved in the department planning process. In a unique application of this process, Conrad Muehling, program director, Pathways Center, and Julie Nathanson, clinical manager, Michiana Rehabilitation Center, pulled together a team composed of staff from their departments to investigate a common issue between the two departments. From casual data collection and a literature search, Muehling found that 60%-70% of head injuries are the result of a chemical dependency. As a clinician, it was painful to watch patients "move through a program where their needs are not met early enough," Mueller said. The team is using the quality planning to design a new rehabilitation-chemical dependency program geared specifically for dual-diagnosis patients, in which patients would be diagnosed and treated by staff from both units. Over the next

Table 3.2. The Department Quality Pl
Process

Step 1: *Key customer(s)*
- Who are your primary internal customers?
- Who are your primary external customers?

Step 2: *Customer requirements*
What requirements, expectations, needs, or standards do you have to meet/exceed for these key customers? (If these are not yet identified, what is your plan for determining what they are? Include this plan under Action Plans.)

Step 3: *Quality indicator(s)*
How do you know how you are doing? What will you monitor to determine whether you are meeting or exceeding requirements/expectations?

Step 4: *Measure(s)*
How will you measure or monitor each quality indicator? What method of data collection will be necessary?

Step 5: *Baseline*
For each quality indicator, what is your present or most recent level of performance? What performance or opportunity gaps are apparent? (If you do not know, what is your plan for establishing a baseline measurement? Include this under "Action plans.")

Step 6: *Goal*
For each indicator what level of performance do you want to achieve during the next period of measurement (month, quarter, year)?

Step 7: *Barriers*
For each customer and/or requirement, what barrier(s) or roadblock(s) do you foresee or presently face (technical, resources, process, policy, and so forth) and what is your plan for dealing with these? (Include your plan under "Action plans.")

Step 8: *Action plans/processes*
For each quality indicator, what actions do you plan to
(a) determine customer requirements?
(b) establish a baseline (if none exists)?
(c) achieve the level of performance you have determined?
(d) deal with existing or anticipated barriers?

Source: *Developed by Memorial Hospital and Health System, South Bend, Indiana. Reprinted with permission.*

everal years, Memorial hopes to tie the budgeting process into the departmental planning process so the two processes are integrated.

Before TQM, each department maintained its own QA plan. As described further in "QA/QI Relationship," the quality plan encompasses QA (that is, quality control) as well as quality planning activities. The requirements and indicators that a department includes in its plan may include performance areas customers do not identify, such as clinical indicators, technical specifications, and professional standards (for example, QA requirements from the Joint Commission). However, because each department must identify and work with its customers, the development of quality plans is encouraging the resolution of problems that QA did not.

For example, in neonatal intensive care, Darla Woodward, clinical coordinator, said that the child birth unit had historically been the most difficult customer. As a result of the department planning process, the two departments are now working on a joint quality plan. They have put together a team to improve the relationship between the units by identifying and meeting each other's requirements. Jon Fouts, program director psychiatry, and his staff began their quality plan by asking the reasons for quality. As mental health professionals, they did not buy the idea that quality was needed to meet third-party requirements. What made TQM stick for them was the possibility of improving care for patients, especially those patients they had not been able to reach in the past. Staff used a visualization technique to help them reach this conclusion and drew a picture of what TQM looked like to them.

Nurses are thriving in the TQM environment at Memorial—they often take the lead in department quality planning and are involved in the numerous QI teams. Two years before Memorial committed to TQM, empowerment was introduced to nurses. In 1986, Susan Crissman, senior vice-president, began offering formal training in empowerment, and all nursing units moved to a shared governing structure in 1987. Each nursing unit elects a unit practice council (UPC), which oversees all the managerial and patient care concerns of the unit (for example, scheduling, QA). On smaller units, the UPC might be made up of all nursing staff. It is up to the UPC whether they want to formulate their unit's quality plan. An elected member from each UPC sits on the organization's nursing council, which looks at organizationwide issues of nursing practice. Two units at Memorial have actually moved into self-governance. Given more responsibility than shared governance units, these two units devise their own budgets and complete performance evaluations.

To Crissman, empowerment not only means providing a fear-free environment, it also involves helping staff improve their self-sufficiency by giving them the skills and resources they need to do their job effectively. The empowerment movement at Memorial was a reaction to the nursing image in the early 1980s. "Nurses suffered from low self-esteem...and were too codependent," Crissman said. A person must believe that his or her "life's work makes a difference...then one begins to enhance [sic] self-esteem," she said. Empowerment at Memorial addresses staff's personal or psychological needs and provides the structure to support it. "You have to have both, " Betz said. "You can't just say we value a person . . . you need to give the structure" to succeed. Memorial's move to shared governance provided this structure.

QI Process

About 25 chartered quality improvement teams (QITs) and many other skunk teams are currently operating at Memorial (see Table 3.3, page 84). Chartered QITs are identified and guided by the Quality Council, which selects the project, drafts a charter, and identifies a "key stakeholder" in the process being evaluated who becomes the team leader. The team leader then works with staff in Mosel's office and the Quality Council advisor to select team members and a facilitator. After the QIT gets underway, members report their recommendations and solutions to the Quality Council for approval. For example, the transportation QIT was charged with "...developing a transportation process which satisfies the needs of patients, families, and the various departments involved." As a result, the team reduced patient waiting time from an average range of 5 to 30 minutes to an average of 4 to 5 minutes, saving an estimated $30,000 annually. (See "QI Supports" for Memorial's cost of quality model.) Jelsma estimates that about 15% of Memorial's work force is involved in chartered QITs. Skunk teams are not directly connected with the Quality Council. Many pop up as the result of department TQM activities. According to Jelsma, most staff who take on skunk work know the process well enough (for example, from being on other chartered QITs) that they need little guidance.

All teams use the same problem-solving approach. After evaluating several approaches, Memorial developed its own process improvement model—IMPROVE—which is a combination of Juran's diagnos-

Table 3.3. A Sample of Memorial's Team Activities

Admitting. Examined entire patient admitting process, including bed control. Enlarged outpatient registration areas and reduced registration wait time to less than five minutes. Provided 24-hour scheduling for catheter lab. Currently implementing centralized scheduling and 1-number admitting for cardiology patients.

Pharmacy Charges. Examined pharmacy charging processes. Identified lost charges on four meds that total over $40,000 annually.

Diabetic Protocol. Developed multidisciplinary critical path for diabetics.

Transportation. Examined inpatient ancillary transportation process. Reduced wait time from an average range of 5–30 minutes to an average of 4–5 minutes for the first quarter of 1991. Improved cost of quality an estimated $30,000 annually.

Rehab Recruitment/Retention. Examined recruitment process and retention practices for professional staff. Reduced recruitment time by 90 days. Improved project cost of quality by $250,000 annually.

Lab Quality Planning. Identified physician requirements for turnaround time on tests and successfully reduced turnaround time to physician's satisfaction.

Neonatal Quality Planning/QI. Improved infant transportation response time as required by referring hospitals. Seventy-five percent of transport responses in less than 30 minutes; satisfaction up 5% (from 73% to 78%) in the first year.

Tissue/Organ Procurement. Internal/external team examined procurement process and documentation. Increased number of donations 300% in first year.

Critical Pathways. Developed critical pathways for home total parenteral nutrition and for total hip/total knee care.

Source: *Developed by Memorial Hospital and Health System, South Bend, Indiana, 1991. Reprinted with permission.*

tic journey approach[3] (steps "I" through "R") and the Shewart cycle (steps "O" through "E"). Figure 3.2 (page 85) illustrates the IMPROVE sequence.

To date the QITs primarily look at administration-related processes. Even though investigating these processes will indirectly affect clinical outcomes, they have not directly addressed questions of clinical effectiveness or efficacy. Currently, Memorial is attacking clinical quality improvement issues through critical pathways, which seeks to move a patient through the hospital system as effectively and

efficiently as possible. For example, Jelsma is working with st[a]
home total parenteral nutrition critical pathway, which

- addresses acceptable length of stay;
- monitors resource utilization;
- incorporates quality management and outcomes to assure quality care;
- promotes collaboration between disciplines; and
- provides opportunity for continuous improvement in the delivery of care through concurrent monitoring.

As a result of the home total parenteral nutrition pathway, Memorial has decreased length of stay (for example, one case saved 21 days or $8,337), physicians now plan admissions with the clinical nurse specialist to coordinate medical and nursing care and "cycle" hyperalimentation earlier in the hospital stay, and patients have improved outcomes (for example, weight gain, no complications or rehospitalizations). Other critical paths now being developed include diabetes, hysterectomy, and coronary artery disease. According to Jelsma, critical paths are chosen by staff interest, internal customers, and data from department quality planning.

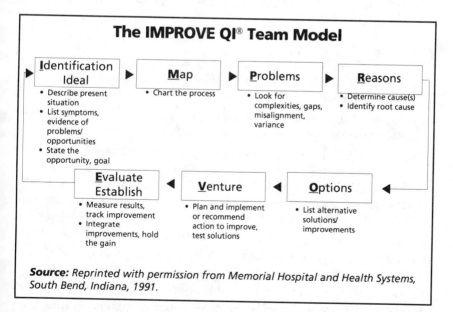

Figure 3.2. Memorial developed its own process improvement model—IMPROVE— which is a combination of Juran's diagnostic journey approach (steps "I" through "R") and the Shewhart cycle (steps "O" through "E").

Since their initial team activities, the Quality Council made several improvements in their methods for selecting projects and chartering teams. For example, they learned from early team experiences that charters that are too large are burdensome. One team was initially asked to look at the entire admitting system and another the entire transportation system. Eventually, the admitting team had to slice the system into different parts and concentrated on it piece by piece. Project selection is now more driven by data than at first. For example, the opportunities identified by staff were quantified and prioritized according to those most frequently mentioned. One team is charted to collect data on a perceived problem in order to determine whether a QIT should be formed. Early activities showed senior management that they are often "out of touch with what happens every day," Mosel said. For example, senior management asked staff to list areas they found problematic in the organization. Prominent on the list were broken equipment, staffing problems, and parking security. Management would never have identified these areas as prominent problems, Newbold said. The Quality Council is also shifting much of the project selection and review process to vice-presidents to drive the QI process further into operations and to free the Council to concentrate on implementation strategy, benchmarking, and macrosystem QI opportunities.

QA/QI Relationship

Since Memorial leans toward Juran, who includes quality control in his trilogy, the decision to integrate QA and TQM is essentially not an issue. While the emphasis is on QI, QA is understood as essential to monitor processes and outcomes to identify improvement opportunities.[3] As discussed earlier, a department's quality plan incorporates QA requirements. This practical approach has provided staff with a simple means to integrate the two processes as well. For example, the Joint Commission requires that all departments (for example, chemical dependency) have a process to monitor the quality of patient care. As part of their department planning process, the chemical dependency service at Memorial must first identify its customers and then the customers' requirements. To meet Joint Commission requirements, the chemical dependency unit identifies the patient as one of its key customers in their quality plan and establishes indicators to monitor those services that are supplied directly or indirectly to the patient. Any other requirements from the Joint Commission, state agencies, and so forth are also included in the plan. Staff simply list them under the section called "requirements." A case study (below) illustrates how the pyschiatric department integrated its QA and QI activities. In addition to reporting to the vice-president on the progress of his or her department's goals, each department director also submits a key indicator report that is distributed to the quality management department; results are incorporated in board QI reports.

Education

The Quality Council decided from the outset that TQM education would begin with management and cascade down through the orga-

(continued on page 93)

Case Study
The Story of Memorial's Psychiatric Quality Improvement Team

Objective

Through our departmental quality planning in Memorial's psychiatric division we hoped to gain an understanding of how traditional quality assurance (QA), which is a retrospective, punishment-oriented way of assuring quality, could be bridged with total quality management (TQM), which is concurrent and finds the root causes of problems to prevent reoccurrence optimally while the patient is still at the hospital.

Need for Quality

The core leadership in psychiatry began by discussing our units' need for quality in any form. We agreed that, first and foremost, as clinicians we have an intrinsic duty to improve the care given to our patients. (We attend educational offerings, belong to networks, and so forth to keep our skills current so that we provide quality care to those who depend on it and expect it.) We also agreed that we needed to incorporate the standards of the Joint Commission and regulators into our department's TQM activities and make them work for us.

After substantiating that it is our obligation to provide quality care, we needed to bridge the gap between the old QA and TQM. We knew we did not want two separate systems to monitor (that is, the TQM plan as well as QA monitors). This sounded like the same old paper chase. At this point we realized that the departmental quality planning process (see Table 3.2, page 85) gave us the tools necessary to map out everything we wanted to accomplish in a clinical setting in an organized fashion. Our QA monitors became key indicators of quality and the

---

"who and how" of the monitoring process fit nicely into the activities.

Monitoring of Clinical Data
We plotted on a flowchart the steps in our departmental planning process (see Figure 3.A, page 89), which included the following:

- Prioritizing and focusing attention on key quality indicators: nursing assessment and psychiatric assessment phases (see Figures 3.B and 3.C, pages 90–91);
- Monitoring these indicators on an ongoing basis and incorporating rotation of all staff disciplines in the monitoring process;
- Discovering points of bias after a trial period:
    — no time frames placed on review process to allow for completion of forms (that is, monitoring to begin after patient is here five to seven days),
    — staff not clear where to locate information in the medical record (that is, monitoring tool did not directly correlate with the medical record), and
    — "yes/no" subject to interpretation (that is, perception bias—whether it objectively meets criteria);
- Developing solutions to improve the process, which included
    — seven-day time frame placed on review process,
    — prompts added to monitor tool to locate information and to correlate directly with assessment format (for example, psychosocial assessment data found under life-style), and
    — "yes/no" format changed to "satisfactory/unsatisfactory" with four descriptive criteria with which to score an unsatisfactory work: not on time, illegible, no signature and/or credentials, and any category with blank spaces;
- Summarizing and presenting nursing information at the monthly QA/TQM leadership meetings and then to the individual units' administrative council meetings for review/action and follow-up with the TQM process; and
- Presenting information pertinent to psychiatrists at monthly psychiatry staff meeting for review and follow-up.

Analysis
After monitoring the indicators, we identified those areas that were a priority for improvement through the use of Pareto analysis, which states that 20% of the causes (the "vital few") account for 80% of the effects. This useful tool helped us concentrate our efforts. When entering our data initially, we input them in the positive (that is, how many times each item occurred in the monitoring process) and discov-

Figure 3.A. Psychiatry's Planning Process

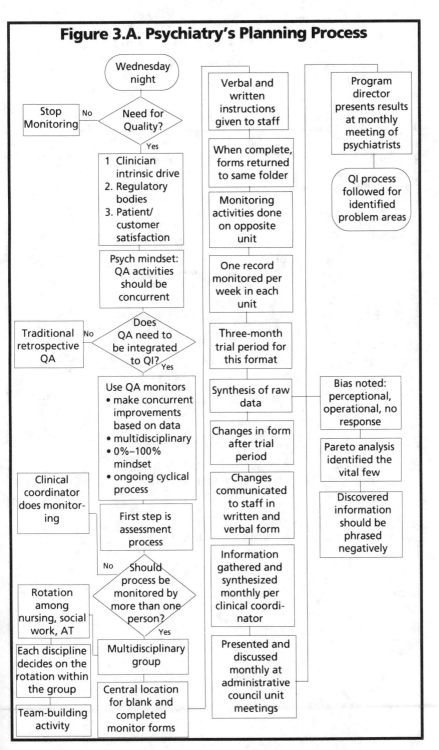

Figure 3.B. Quality Assurance Chart Review— Assessment Phase

Medical Record # _____ Admission Date _____
Physician _____ Date of Review _____

The Nursing Assessment	N/A	Yes	No
Completed by an RN within 24 hours	___	___	___
Contains: Physical characteristics	___	___	___
Functional characteristics	___	___	___
Psychosocial characteristics	___	___	___
Past/current medical history	___	___	___
Patient/family education needs	___	___	___
Discharge planning needs	___	___	___
Environment/equipment needs	___	___	___
Patient status at time of arrival	___	___	___
Strengths and liabilities	___	___	___
The patient's primary is identified within 24 hours	___	___	___

The Psychiatric Evaluation	N/A	Yes	No
Completed by a psychiatrist within 60 hours (N/A to HOPE)	___	___	___
Contains: Working diagnosis	___	___	___
Chief complaint	___	___	___
History of present illness	___	___	___
Mental status exam			
Behavioral problem	___	___	___
Legal concerns when present	___	___	___
Initial goal for beginning treatment			
Nutritional assessment (HOPE only)	___	___	___
A history and physical is completed within 24 hours	___	___	___
A social history is completed by the fifth day	___	___	___
An AT/RT assessment is completed by the fifth day	___	___	___

Psychological/neurological tests (newly diagnosed
patients or all HOPE patients)   ___ ___ ___

_____
Reviewer's signature

90

Figure 3.C. Quality Improvement Chart Review— Assessment Phase

Review date _____

Patient name _____

Medical record # _____

Admission date _____

Physician _____

Unsatisfactory is defined as
1. not on time
2. illegible
3. no signature and or credentials
4. any category with blank spaces

Key
Satisfactory = X
Unsatisfactory = 1, 2, 3, 4

Nursing Assessment	Satisfactory	Unsatisfactory
Completed by an RN within 4 hours*		
Contains: Psychosocial (life-style)		
Medical history		
Physical assessment		
Functional characteristics		
Environment/equipment needs (ADLs)		
Strengths and liabilities		
Patient/family education needs		
Patient status at time of arrival (initial entry in nursing notes)		

The Psychiatric Evaluation	Satisfactory	Unsatisfactory
Completed by a psychiatrist within 60 hours (located on admission history form, progress note, or consult sheet)		
Contains: Chief complaint		
Reason for admission		
Admitting evaluation (violent, suicidal, and so on)		
History of present illness		
Mental status exam		
Previous psych treatment		
Reason outpatient not appropriate		
Family history		
Social history		
Provisional diagnosis (per DSMIIIR)		
Estimated length of stay		
Provisional discharge plan		

Comments:

History and Physical completed in 24 hours
Assessment completed by fifth day
Social history completed by fifth day

ered that our statistical process results did not match the initial analysis of our raw data. We then entered the data from the negative standpoint (how many times each item was not found during the monitoring process) and found that the results were compatible with the findings of the raw data. This was a valuable lesson learned for future data collection (see Figures 3.D, below, and 3.E, page 93).

Conclusion

This information led to enhancements of the assessment process for nursing in the department of psychiatry to include separate flowsheets for medication and health teaching as well as a stronger integration of discharge planning into the initial assessment and treatment plan. These enhancements are a part of quality nursing care as much as Joint Commission and Board of Health requirements.

Revisions in the process for psychiatric assessment were also initiated. A specific history/physical format was developed for the department of psychiatry as well as a detailed psychiatric evaluation form that met the criteria outlined by the Board of Health. This information, as well as social histories and legal status, are being monitored daily by the night shift staff, and any discrepancies are being followed by the nurse manager.

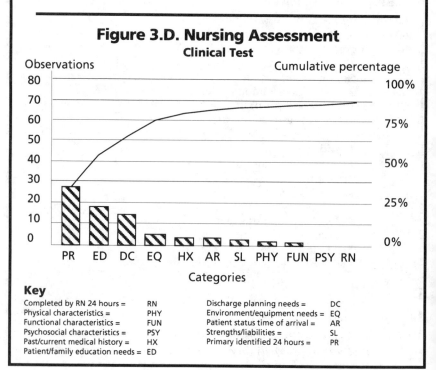

Figure 3.D. Nursing Assessment
Clinical Test

Key

Completed by RN 24 hours =	RN
Physical characteristics =	PHY
Functional characteristics =	FUN
Psychosocial characteristics =	PSY
Past/current medical history =	HX
Patient/family education needs =	ED

Discharge planning needs =	DC
Environment/equipment needs =	EQ
Patient status time of arrival =	AR
Strengths/liabilities =	SL
Primary identified 24 hours =	PR

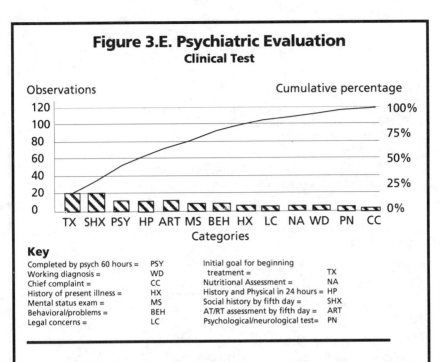

Figure 3.E. Psychiatric Evaluation
Clinical Test

Key

Completed by psych 60 hours =	PSY	Initial goal for beginning	
Working diagnosis =	WD	treatment =	TX
Chief complaint =	CC	Nutritional Assessment =	NA
History of present illness =	HX	History and Physical in 24 hours =	HP
Mental status exam =	MS	Social history by fifth day =	SHX
Behavioral/problems =	BEH	AT/RT assessment by fifth day =	ART
Legal concerns =	LC	Psychological/neurological test=	PN

Another quality tool we found useful in the clinical area was flow-charting, which we utilized in the process of initially setting up our partial hospitalization program.

Source: *The case study was developed by Denise Wynegar, RN, Clinical Coordinator Behavioral Health, of Memorial's Psychiatric Division, 1991. Reprinted with permission. Members of the team included Jon Fouts, MSW, CTRS, Program Director Psychiatry; Nancy Jelsma, MSN, RN, CNA, Clinical Quality Specialist; and Denise Wynegar.*

(continued from page 87)

nization. Top and middle management have received extensive education (7.5 days formal training) in TQM concepts, tools, quality planning, and teamwork during their annual retreats. While all employees have received an eight-hour awareness course (which took two years to provide to all staff), most tool training is provided on a just-in-time basis for QITs and departments developing their quality plans. Table 3.4 (page 94) provides a summary of training provided at Memorial to date. While this method may have slowed the deployment of TQM knowledge through the organization, management elected this method out of concern that providing staff with a lot of training without the resources available to support them (that is, facilitators,

Table 3.4. Memorial's Training Rollout: The First Three Years

Management Education:

Year 1 (1989)—2.5 days led by the Quality Council
- Quality concepts/awareness (ODI course)
- Quality through People structure—2 tracks
- Roles of managers in TQM

Year 2 (1990)—2.5 days led by facilitators
Training shifted to tools in the second year to make process work
- Basic five tools
- IMPROVE
- Department quality planning
- Teamwork skills

Year 3 (1991)
- Advanced tools
- Process refinements
- Quality planning
- Cultural diversity

Staff Education:

Eight-hour course taught by the Quality Council. Everyone will have received the course by August 1991
- Concepts
- Team training (IMPROVE)
- Department quality planning
- Empowerment

Physician Education:

Beginning in 1991, an overview of TQM concepts and QI tools for medical staff officers was provided to physicians.

Source: Developed by Memorial Hospital and Health System, South Bend, Indiana. Reprinted with permission.

management direction) would leave staff "all dressed up with nowhere to go," Mosel said. Management expects that the department planning process will provide an avenue for all staff to become involved in TQM until they can provide them with more training. Looking back, Memorial would have provided each department with more guidance during the planning process since the departments that did best "did so with the help of a facilitator who essentially walked them through" the process, Mosel said.

While they adapted awareness materials from ODI, Mosel and his staff have developed the rest of Memorial's curriculum, including a four-day facilitator course. Quality Council members participate in teaching the introductory sessions for managers and staff.

As discussed in "Strategy," empowerment classes were offered to all nurses beginning in 1986.

QI Supports

Tied closely to Memorial's TQM effort has been building a strong support system that ensures comprehensive customer feedback, recognizes teams for their accomplishments, provides process-oriented data to teams, and so forth.

Customer-supplier feedback: As discussed earlier, Memorial was doing customer research before TQM. "All research did not directly fall out of TQM," Teri Russo, director of marketing information said, "but it got renewed life with TQM. . . . [TQM] has fostered a mentality throughout the organization to find out more about customers." Early in the hospital's TQM activities, management identified five key customers of the organization: patients, physicians, payers, public (for example, health care consumers, media), and employees. Russo lists several methods they are using to obtain feedback from all these groups:

- *Patient satisfaction survey.* After discharge, patients are mailed a survey. Developed by Press-Ganey, a local market research company, the surveys are tied to a data base that includes 180 other hospitals. Memorial is able to compare its own performance over time and against health care organizations that are like Memorial (that is, same demographics). The organizationwide and department-specific quality goals may be determined from the survey, except in departments that are not directly linked to patient care or where the scores might be heavily weighted by patient biases (for example, intensive care, because patients may not remember their stay). When departments want more specific or additional information, they often design their own surveys. Departments are encouraged to funnel these studies through marketing.

- *Focus group research.* Between 40 and 50 focus groups were held in 1990 compared to the 5 usually held each year before TQM. All 5 key customer groups were reached. Memorial has its own focus group facility on-site that has a one-way mirror, and a trained moderator always facilitates each focus group. The data collected from these groups provide management with much more in-depth feedback on the issues that the Press-Ganey survey identified.

- *Community image study.* Each year, Memorial conducts a random telephone survey of people in the community. They ask such questions as "which hospital stands out with highest quality?" The 20-25 minute survey provides the organization with specific feedback on its image throughout the community.

- *Interviews with and surveys of physicians.* Administrators continually conduct one-on-one interviews with the key admitters among Memorial's medical staff. Staff are also finalizing a survey that will hit all medical staff members, not only key admitters.

- *Staff opinion survey.* Conducted biannually, the survey provides staff with an opportunity to express their opinions and ideas. Questions range from "My pay is enough to give me a reasonable amount of security" to "I understand Quality Through People."

Reflecting on Memorial's history of customer service, Newbold says inpatient satisfaction scores have consistently been in the 80s on the Press-Ganey survey (100 being the highest on the scale). Frustrated, senior management decided to respond directly to patient complaints for 120 days. As soon as a complaint was reported, a vice-president went to the patient's room and took care of the complaint. However, after this period, the satisfaction score was still ranked in the 80s. Newbold learned that true customer satisfaction exists when the patient never has a chance to complain because the nurse, attending physician, or other staff member fixes the problem before the patient becomes upset enough to complain. Newbold figures he will know a true culture change has occurred at Memorial when customer service is so ingrained that line staff respond to customer needs immediately.

Information services. With access to a data base that includes clinical data, patient demographics, procedure volumes, and diagnostic-related group information, staff are able to retrieve most information they need for TQM activities. Each patient care unit has one terminal, which is connected to a Hewlett-Packard minicomputer. There are also 100 personal computers within the organization. Staff from information services will design special programs to assist QITs to collect and display data, according to Marty Lebbin, director of management services. Facilitators and teams also have access to software packages that can be used to develop control charts and other TQM tools, including one personal computer that is dedicated to support of clinical QI efforts.

As part of their affiliation with the Voluntary Hospitals of America, Memorial participates in two comparative data systems:

- *Data Comparison Reporting System (DCRS).* This system provides comparative data in such areas as work hours, paid hours, patient hours, and so forth. Lebbin compares DCRS to Monitrend. Department heads use this information for benchmarking and may receive several types of comparative reports (for example, by region, by hospital size).

- *Clinical/Financial Information System (CFIS).* Although not fully implemented yet, this integrated clinical and financial data system will provide comparative data tracking across 100–150 diagnostic-related groups for use in QA/QI.

Lebbin hopes to provide for physician access to more information in the future: The Voluntary Hospitals of America is setting up (via their local tristate area) an electronic library that physicians can access to conduct private studies.

Reward and recognition. Quality is tied to compensation for the entire management staff. Their performance evaluations and salaries depend significantly on their department's quality and financial goals, according to Virginia Chism, vice-president, human resources. The quality goal is arrived at from patient satisfaction scores and the department quality plan. The patient satisfaction score comes from the patient survey conducted.

Steve Birchard, vice-president, found that the managers of the support departments he oversees need the same type of outside motivation. Because the support departments (for example, materials management, food service) are not tied directly to patient care, the managers' salaries are not determined directly by the quality score. The departments were "not getting anywhere" with their department plans, Birchard said, until he initiated monthly meetings. Support department managers now gather to report on and help each other develop their plans, which has successfully placed positive peer pressure on department managers. Birchard is also developing a comparable measure to the quality score for nonclinical departments.

To provide further incentive to managers, Memorial has begun a shared bonus plan. When the organization meets its annual financial and quality goals (see "Strategy" section), management will divide a financial bonus among those managers who satisfactorily met their goals that year. Eventually, Chism hopes to develop similar programs for all employees.

Recognition for participation in QI activities is also done indirectly through quarterly Quality Forums where teams present QI projects, reports to the Quality Council, and the weekly newsletter.

Suppliers. Currently, Memorial treats staff from contractual organizations as Memorial employees, not "X Company" employees, according to Birchard. For example, the department manager of nutritional services (a Marriott employee) is required to develop a quality plan just like other departments. Memorial's contractual agreement with Marriott is linked to the quality goals set by nutritional services in their department quality plan. Staff also participate in performance evaluations and receive TQM training at Memorial's expense. Some Marriott employees have even been trained as facilitators.

Birchard is also using TQM concepts to improve relationships with product suppliers. He hopes to establish performance agreements that require a quarterly performance monitoring system based on quality indicators. When bidding, a product supplier would have to include quality criteria as well as cost estimates, which will allow purchase decisions to be based more on quality than price.

Memorial has begun to include suppliers in team activities. The organ procurement team includes two staff people from the organ banks.

Cost-of-quality measurement. Memorial developed its own cost-of-quality measurement to help team members see the financial impact of the solutions they propose. As shown in Figure 3.3 (page 99) the model firsts asks the team to determine the operating costs of the process before improvement (for example, poor outpatient transportation systems were costing Memorial $55,500 annually in overtime, lost revenue, and so on) and then to project the future costs of the improved process (for example, $25,000 in additional staff, time spent in quality planning). The team will then be able to determine the amount of money saved (that is, a $30,500 difference between present and projected costs) by the improvement they suggest.[4] Mike Koziol, vice-president for finance, said Memorial elected this simple model over one that also factors in the constant operating costs involved in a process, such as staff training and direct operating costs. From a financial point of view, the more complex model would have provided "a more accurate financial picture of the total investment in quality," Koziol said, but from a practical standpoint it would prove to be "too in-depth for the average manager." One of the main purposes of the model is to emphasize cost-effectiveness to staff. According to Newbold, many initial teams suggested adding benefits and resources (that is,

Memorial's Cost of Quality Analysis Worksheet

	Department A	Department B	Total
A. Present Cost			
Staff	$35,500		$35,500
Equipment			
Supplies			
Other	20,000		20,000
Subtotal	55,500		55,500
B. Proposed Cost			
Staff	18,500		18,500
Equipment			
Supplies			
Other	6,500		6,500
Subtotal	25,000		25,000
C. A – B	30,500		30,500
D. Revenue Gain	20,000		20,000
E. Cost of Quality Improvement (A – B) + D	50,500		50,500
Percentage Improvement E/A	90.99%		

Source: Developed by Memorial Hospital and Health System, South Bend, IN, 1991. Reprinted with permission.

Figure 3.3. Teams at Memorial used this cost-of-quality analysis worksheet to help see the financial impact of the solutions they propose.

building a new parking lot) before eliminating rework. "It's a lot more sexy to build a new parking lot," Newbold said. The Quality Council eventually had to stress that it would be very difficult to get new full-time employees as a result of team activities.

Benchmarking. Memorial has been involved in extensive benchmarking from the very beginning of its TQM effort. Recently, staff have started targeting their benchmarking to specific areas of interest. For example, staff attended Motorola University, in Schaumburg, Illinois, to look specifically at their training process and investigated Xerox's performance rewards system. Memorial is also a member of the Healthcare Forum's Quality Improvement Network, the VHA Tri-State network and, through the Healthcare Forum, the

American Productivity Center's National Benchmarking Clearing-house project.

Physician Involvement

Memorial decided to lay some groundwork before extensively involv-ing the medical staff in the TQM effort. During the last few years, they have concentrated on enlisting the support of physician leaders and targeting TQM improvements that successfully saved physician time or made their job easier (for example, improving turnaround for emergency room lab tests). According to Bob White, MD, director, neonatal intensive care unit, it is important for hospitals moving toward TQM to recruit physician leaders early in the effort, not only elected leaders but also those he refers to as "Don Quixote types," or those who are activists, because "they will identify the issues that need to be addressed." White was one of the Don Quixote types senior management identified. They "came to me and said here's your chance to make a difference," White remembers. Stacking up TQM successes that directly affect physicians will help prove that TQM is not another fad. White said that physicians are "not as interested in costs as improved outcomes." However, "if cerebral palsy outcomes im-prove because TQM identified three ways to do things better, physi-cians will be really curious," he said.

Besides physician leaders, many physicians at Memorial have become involved in TQM through department quality planning, participating on QITs, and strategic quality planning/visioning. Memorial is plan-ning to begin involving physicians on a wider scale in the near future and provide more training. A new position, senior vice-president, medical staff, was recently created. In this position, Jim Hoffman, MD, will help roll out TQM among the medical staff; he projects 10–14 medical staff projects in 1992. White estimates that in three years 50% of medical staff will be involved.

Various medical staff and organizational leaders identified several barriers involved in recruiting physicians to TQM:

- Many physicians have trouble seeing themselves as part of a system. "Physicians don't see the 40 some steps to get medication back to the patient . . . they're taken away from the systems approach," White said.
- It is necessary to provide good data and information to physicians. Much of the data physicians obtain through QA and case review

does not provide them with any information they do not already know. Alan Snell, MD, a family practitioner, hopes to see physicians become more involved in data management. "We need to get to the level where physicians can . . . manipulate data, regroup it in ways so it helps them," he said. The medical staff hopes the recent purchase of MEDISGROUPS will help in this process. Eventually, Snell would like to be able to use data to look across the entire episode of illness.

- Time is precious. The medical staff at Memorial agree that available time for physicians to participate in TQM training and activities is a problem. However, one physician claimed he would be pleased to monitor projects that gave him useful data.

- Many physicians live in a false paradise. Memorial has a "really complacent group of physicians," White said. "They may not feel there is much that needs fixing. The perception is that most of the problems are in the big city . . . the nice thing about practicing in Indiana is we're a long way away from that." While admitting this is a false paradise, White stresses that "perception is as important as reality."

Conclusion

Memorial is confident that TQM will enable the hospital to meet the challenges facing health care. Mosel predicts that the next ten years will test health care "like the last ten years didn't begin to." But according to Newbold, "If we stay focused on quality, have good outcomes, processes . . . what difference does it make what happens in [Washington] DC?" Akin to a good sports team that can easily adjust to the goal line being pushed back, Newbold believes "a good organization that is involved in TQM doesn't have to worry about external pressures. They have the processes in place to address any issue that comes up." Far from being intimidated by the future, staff and board members are challenging themselves with their vision of Memorial in the year 2000.

References

1. Peters T: *Thriving on Chaos.* New York: Harper & Row, 1987, pp 322–323.

2. Senge PM: *The Fifth Discipline.* New York: Doubleday/Currency, 1990.

3. Juran JM: *Juran on Planning for Quality*. New York: The Free Press, 1988.

4. Newbold PA, Mosel D: Quality through people: Integrating budgeting, strategic planning, and quality management. *The Quality Letter*, Nov 1990, pp 8–13.

4 Anchoring the Community

Magic Valley Regional Medical Center
Twin Falls, Idaho

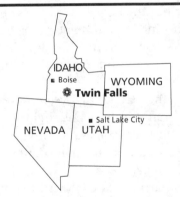

Type of hospital: Community medical center owned by the county

Scope of services: General medical/surgical

Beds: 165, with average census of 72

Extent of CQI involvement: Since a commitment in 1988, management has identified the "anchoring" of the hospital board as the most vital accomplishment of their rollout to date. The strengths of their CQI effort lie in their vision—"to make Magic Valley the healthiest place in America"— and the community's involvement in achieving that vision

Special aspects of Magic Valley's CQI activities:
— Communitywide involvement
— An "anchored" hospital board
— Outside groups used to leverage internal change
— Vision to "make Magic Valley the healthiest place in America"
— Internal infrastructure that supports move to CQI and includes organizational visioning, a new computer system, integration of QA/QI, nursing clinical practice model, and revamped compensation system

Although Magic Valley Regional Medical Center is the smallest hospital profiled in this publication, with an average census of 72 patients, its continuous quality improvement (CQI) activities encompass the community of Twin Falls and the surrounding four counties in southern Idaho. When senior management and the board sat down to reexamine the hospital's vision in the context of Deming's philosophy, they realized that if the hospital was going to make a significant difference in providing health care, they would have to build a cooperative effort that addressed all the parts of the system that keeps a patient healthy, including preventive health care and education. "Health care is not doing well by having narrow boundaries," says John Bingham, administrator, and suggests it is time to consider "wider boundaries." The hospital's vision is to "be a standard of excellence and cooperation in making Magic Valley the healthiest place in America." To achieve this vision the hospital is working on two levels: building a strong infrastructure within the walls of the hospital to support the transition to CQI and facilitating a communitywide effort to improve the health of its citizens using CQI methods. This effort will involve the competing hospital, city government, local businesses, the junior college, and others. The link between internal and external efforts is the hospital board. Bingham and his senior management have spent the past two years "anchoring" the board in the concepts of CQI and the hospital's vision. Anchoring is an understanding and commitment to CQI that results in a sense of ownership. Bingham believes a board that has internalized these concepts will in turn anchor the hospital and the community.

Two-and-a-half years after beginning their CQI initiative, most staff and a large number of people in the community have bought into the concepts of CQI and are beginning to speak the same language. Successes are being won on both fronts. Internally, management is using CQI methods and tools as though they are second nature. Teams have begun to show successes, and departmental CQI activities are helping to break down barriers across departments and disciplines. As a result of the examples the hospital is providing, local businesses, city government, and others have begun to believe that the hospital is serious about a communitywide effort. For instance, Magic Valley invited key players in the community, including competing hospitals, to a CQI seminar at no cost. The hospital also used its funds to recruit several specialty physicians to the area after identifying that a number one concern in Twin Falls was the recruitment of physicians. More telling than these initial successes, however, is the determination voiced by Bingham, his senior management, and the board. Although conscious of the long road ahead, Bingham does not flinch when speaking about making "Magic Valley the healthiest place in America."

Description and Demographics

With a population of 27,500, Twin Falls is the largest city in an eight-county area in south central Idaho known as Magic Valley, which is surrounded on all sides by either mountains or desert. The rich and famous have been vacationing in the Magic Valley area for years, specifically in nearby Sun Valley on the edge of the Sawtooth Mountains, which provides skiing and other recreational escapes. For the people who live in the area year-round, however, agriculture is the mainstay. Irrigation has turned land that was essentially nonfarmable into one million acres of some of the most productive farmland in the country. Potatoes, sugar beets, corn, vegetable seeds, barley, beans, grass seeds, oats, and hay are the predominant crops. Fish farming (85% of the nation's commercially-raised trout come from Magic Valley) and dairy farming are important industries as well. Due to the trend toward fewer and larger farms across the country, employment growth is beginning to shift from agriculture to the trade and service industries. The abundance of natural resources has brought a substantial number of food processing companies to the region, including Green Giant, Pet, Kraft, Ore-Ida Foods, Del Monte, Coors, Amalgamated Sugar, and Universal Foods, which is the largest employer in the region. The economy of the area has been consistently slow and stable and has not yet been affected by the recent recession.

Magic Valley is a 165-bed facility owned by Twin Falls County. Although county-owned, Magic Valley is self-sufficient and has not had to request tax dollar support since 1978. The hospital is helped in part by its "arm's length" relationship with the Magic Valley Regional Medical Center Foundation, a nonprofit organization established to raise funds for health-related activities. Magic Valley has a financial advantage over many other public hospitals; the area has a low percentage of fixed reimbursement patients (50% Medicare patients, low number of HMOs and PPOs). Magic Valley provides medical, surgical, pediatric, and obstetrical services primarily to residents of Twin Falls, Jerome, and Gooding Counties. However, Magic Valley's service area stretches beyond these three counties, and the hospital has been designated by Medicare as a rural referral center. The patient population is lower-middle class and moderately educated with generally positive health characteristics. More ambulatory and emergency room patients are usually present on a given day at Magic Valley than inpatients. However, the medical center recently opened a cancer center, which has caused an influx of inpatients. The medical staff includes 120 physicians of whom 73 are active; these physicians represent 19 specialty areas.

Several linkages have assisted the medical center in its movement toward CQI. Like Parkview Episcopal Medical Center, Magic Valley is managed by Quorum Health Resources, formerly the management company of Hospital Corporation of America (HCA). As part of their contract, HCA provided, and now Quorum provides, the hospital with educational materials, consultation, and networking opportunities. Magic Valley has also received considerable support from the companies located in the area that have strong CQI initiatives in place, particularly Universal Foods, which invites hospital staff and others in the community to CQI seminars.

History

Bingham felt health care administration provided a good avenue for him to "give back what he takes out" of society. He feels hospital administrators, like physicians, have spheres of influence inside and outside the organization, which allow them to serve as catalysts for change. However, it was not until he began reading about CQI several years ago that he found a method for making such a change. Excited by the ideas and methodologies of W. Edwards Deming, he asked HCA if he could be involved in any activities they initiated involving CQI; Magic Valley eventually became one of HCA's pilot hospitals for CQI.

Although Bingham introduced CQI to Magic Valley in late 1988, he does not date the official start of their CQI initiative until October 1989. Believing at first that all you needed was a core group of employees educated in CQI to begin a cultural change, Bingham began training staff and board members up front. A Quality Improvement Council (QIC), which includes all senior management, was formed to direct the rollout. Teams sprang up, but "several failed miserably at first," Bingham said. Although they used CQI tools, they did not "understand work as process, statistical thinking," or other CQI concepts. More importantly, Bingham believes they were "not anchored, not grounded in understanding the philosophical vision of the organization." A lull ensued, due in large part to the fact that Magic Valley had simply adopted the generic guiding principles HCA provided. Eventually the QIC "realized they didn't understand what these meant"; they had not internalized the meaning of the guidelines.

In the fall of 1989, the QIC decided to temporarily slow down training. Senior management and the board concentrated on formulating a strategy that would support the move to CQI both internally and externally. This included

- an "anchored" senior management and board;
- a hospital vision and CQI strategy that was unique to Magic Valley; and
- an infrastructure that addressed theoretical and practical issues of applying CQI techniques at the medical center.

Senior management agree that the time they took to anchor themselves and the board was one of the most vital parts of their rollout. An anchored board and senior management mean not only that they are educated in and understand the hospital's new direction, but also that they have internalized and are committed to this direction. Anchoring is not a strict, step-by-step approach; different methods may work. For example, senior management and board members at Magic Valley rewrote Deming's 14 points to apply to the medical center and taught CQI methods and tools to others. Key to the anchoring process at Magic Valley was the development of a hospital vision and strategy for CQI implementation. As explained further in the "Philosophy" and "Strategy" sections, the board's strategic planning committee envisioned Magic Valley's future and is devising a strategy to help the medical center reach this vision.

The hospital's emphasis on planning enabled the QIC and board to address important theoretical and practical issues that might have impeded the rollout of CQI in the hospital up front. For example, they formulated a plan to integrate quality assurance (QA) and CQI, devised a computer system that allows the collection of process-oriented data, adopted a nursing clinical practice model that supports a nursing process-dominated practice, and eliminated their merit pay system. Each of these changes to the infrastructure is addressed in more detail throughout the chapter.

Presently Magic Valley is completing the first phase of the rollout plan it adopted from HCA and Quorum, (see Figure 4.1, page 108) and is continuing to implement CQI among staff and physicians. Department managers and their staff have begun identifying their customers and the processes important to these customers. Because the QIC concentrated first on anchoring themselves and the board and on formulating the strategy and infrastructure needed for their CQI implementation, the rollout to staff and physicians will have a strong foundation.

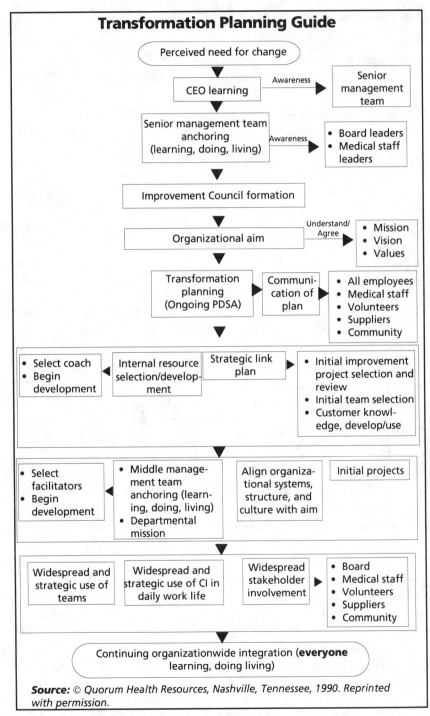

Figure 4.1. Magic Valley has adopted Quorum's rollout plan for CQI.

Philosophy

In formulating the hospital's vision, many members of the board's strategic planning committee brought experiences of attempting to improve a system by concentrating on only one of its parts. Paul Miles, MD, a pediatrician on the medical staff as well as a board member, has been working with the Idaho State Perinatal Project to "make Idaho the healthiest place to have a baby." After first determining that the proper equipment improved the outcome of pregnancy, the state perinatal project worked to ensure that the correct equipment was used in delivery rooms across the state. However, despite their efforts, neonatal mortality rates remained the same. Providing the proper care during the mother's stay in the hospital was not enough to improve mortality rates. The clinic had no control over what happened before and after the hospital stay, Miles said. This experience correlated with the systems thinking Deming promotes.

An understanding of the concepts of collaborative efforts and systems working within larger systems caused the board to realize that medical care provided at Magic Valley was only one component of the health care system in the community. To truly improve care, the committee decided to widen the boundaries of the hospital's efforts to encompass the entire community and to expand the hospital's scope of care to encompass prevention as well as treatment. When the board put the framework together, its vision was that the hospital "will be a standard of excellence and cooperation in making Magic Valley the healthiest place in America." Integral to this vision are four key concepts the board identified:

- *Leadership.* Being proactive in seeking solutions to community health issues;

- *Quality.* Striving for excellence through continuous improvement of services, mindful of the needs of the primary customer— the patient;

- *Collaboration.* Seeking opportunities to work with other providers and organizations to improve the health status of area residents; and

- *Community.* Relying on a broad understanding of community and recognition of community interdependence with respect to health care system development.

To carry out their vision the board has begun to identify major disease categories the community might address first and has developed a model to guide its efforts. After studying public health data, including mortality and morbidity indicators provided by the Idaho Hospital Association, they identified accident prevention as one area the community could affect. Public health data show that accidents are the fourth leading cause of death in Idaho and that Twin Falls is the second most dangerous Idaho city in which to drive; 20% of the hospital's admissions to pediatrics are the result of an auto accident. Other areas identified are heart disease and cancer, which are the first and second causes of death in Idaho, respectively. To address these areas, the board and senior staff developed a six-step circular model, based on public health concepts, which encompasses education, prevention, screening, diagnosis, treatment, and rehabilitation. Bingham describes the model as "an organizational template for assessment."

For example, Miles and others on the board have begun to extensively apply the model to cancer. As part of this model, they held a free prostate screening for the community with funds from a $½ million donation. Seven hundred men showed up for the free screening, and 70 potential cancers were identified and referred for further screening. They hope to offer free colon screening in the near future. The hospital has begun applying the six-step model to heart disease and accident prevention as well. As part of the program for accident prevention, the hospital has formed a coalition within the community that is attempting to reduce accidents in Twin Falls and is teaching accident prevention to parents of all pediatrics patients.

The hospital defines a transformed organization by the degree of focus it places on benefiting society (see Table 4.1, page 111). Bingham stresses that it is a "sense of contribution that makes people become involved." Bingham believes that hospitals have the opportunity to enlist people's need to contribute to a larger end. "It's hard to have a passion for potatoes, but a lot easier to have a passion for helping kids," Bingham said. Magic Valley's emphasis on holistic health is wide enough in scope to involve each person in the community and far-reaching enough to provide a challenge. The direction Magic Valley is taking adheres in large part to Deming with strong influences from Senge[1] and Bronowski.[2] Bingham believes Magic Valley's approach is in concert with Deming's emphasis on systems thinking. The combination of CQI methods and a vision aimed at benefiting society has proven successful so far in recruiting staff and others in the community to their mission. The emphasis on systems thinking and customer-

Table 4.1. Magic Valley's Parameters of a Transformed Organization

1. Degree of focus on benefitting society
   - Vision statement focus
   - Reason for pursuing CQI
   - Alignment of daily work life with vision statement

2. Pervasiveness of a continuous improvement culture

• Board	How well staff understand
• Medical staff	• 14 obligations
• Department activities	• Statistical thinking
• Daily work life	• Systems thinking
	• Scientific method
	• Hoshin-type planning

3. Intensity of joy in work
   - Intrinsic motivation
   - Opportunity to achieve potential
   - Involvement in making a higher contribution to the world

Source: Developed by Magic Valley Regional Medical Center, Twin Falls, Idaho, 1990. Reprinted with permission.

supplier relationships made Universal Foods and other businesses and individuals more appreciative of the interdependence of roles within the community. Judy Robinett, a board member, does not believe her employer, Universal Foods, would have been "so apt to join ranks with the medical center" before the company made its own move to CQI.

Strategy

Bingham feels they have "come a long way from the competitive model" that hospitals across the country have practiced. Bingham and members of Magic Valley's board appear genuinely uncomfortable with language that suggests a competitive approach. For example, several years ago the board envisioned that the medical center would become "a regional force" in health care. Bingham no longer feels the word *force* is "conducive to the collaborative approach" they are fostering in Twin Falls. Miles emphasizes that they are trying to leave competitiveness behind for the sake of a communitywide, holistic approach to health. In contrast to the hospital edging out its competitors, Magic Valley wants to use CQI as the catalyst to bring competitors and the community together. Staff at Magic Valley see CQI more as the method to reach their vision than as an end.

The structure of Magic Valley's CQI activities is key to the success of its strategy. The board appointed a strategic planning committee in October 1989 to oversee the strategy for rolling out CQI both in the hospital and community. To achieve the vision of "making Magic Valley the healthiest place in America," the committee identified five strategic areas for the hospital to concentrate on and appointed subcommittees focusing on the following:

- *Quality.* The subcommittee is concentrating on building the quality framework needed to implement CQI throughout the community, including formulating the model for vision discussed on page 109 and developing measures of the hospital's success. Recently, the subcommittee has been working with the Chamber of Commerce to institute training for the business community in the Twin Falls area.

- *Services.* Subcommittee members are developing five key program areas for the hospital and community to focus on, based on identified community need. The subcommittee's first priority has been the recruitment of physicians for the entire community, which was identified as a concern by hospital customers. As discussed earlier, Magic Valley used hospital funds to recruit five specialty physicians to the area.

- *External Relations.* Charged with collaborating and developing strong relationships with the eight Magic Valley counties, the subcommittee initiated formation of a regional council to better meet the medical needs of Magic Valley and northern Nevada and achieve the medical center's vision.

- *Human Resources.* Concentrating on broadening the employee base and devising ways to "value" hospital staff, the subcommittee is determining recruitment and recognition possibilities.

- *Fiscal Resources and Physical Plant.* The subcommittee is developing a master facilities plan (plant and equipment) that will ensure adequate fiscal and plant resources to achieve Magic Valley's vision.

The subcommittees that were appointed to roll out each of these focus areas include representatives from the community, board, and hospital. For example, the services subcommittee includes the executive director of the Chamber of Commerce, several members of the medical staff, an associate professor from the College of Southern

Idaho, several board members, Bingham, and Jim Murphy, assistant administrator. This mix not only ensures that the views of all parties are considered, but also helps enlist the community in the hospital's efforts and spreads CQI methodologies throughout the various segments. CQI tools and meeting management techniques are used at all subcommittee meetings. As discussed further under "QI Supports," customer feedback along with mortality/morbidity data help direct the decisions made by the strategic planning committee and the five subcommittees.

Although not fully developed, the quality subcommittee is investigating the development of a "vision index," which will allow the hospital to measure how well the community's health is improving. These measures will be linked to the top causes for morbidity/mortality over the past five years in the Magic Valley region, which ties back to the six-step model being developed for improvements in cancer, accident prevention, and heart disease. Eventually, indicators that measure these areas will be developed and shared with the community. Among the indicators being considered for the vision index are infant mortality, neonatal mortality, mothers with prenatal care, immunization rate, seat belt use, and percentage of smokers. "For a hospital to function, you have to have outcome data," Miles said. "But if you look just at outcome data for the hospital . . . you miss out on the bigger issues." He uses the cancer treatment center as an example. Staff might monitor outcomes and death rates for the cancer center over a five-year period, which indicates that the center's survival rate is improving. But at the same time, the community's mortality rate for cancer could be rising, and they would not be "meeting community needs," Miles said.

As senior management and the board complete the hospitalwide strategy for CQI, middle management and staff are beginning to implement CQI within their own spheres through their department rollout activities. Magic Valley is beginning to roll out CQI systematically through all the departments. As part of this, each department is expected to identify its customers and the processes important to those customers. These activities often lead to possibilities for improvement. For example, after collecting data on a process their customers had identified as broken, staff in business services discovered a problem in billing for IVs. Using problem-solving techniques, staff investigated the problem and instituted solutions.

Many staff saw CQI as a fad in the beginning. "The first question they asked was 'What if Bingham leaves?'" said Sharon Fischer, quality resources director. And the second question was "Is the hospital board committed?" For department managers and staff to trust that CQI is not just a fad, Bingham believes "the program should fit the doctrine." For example, he stresses that Magic Valley's budget should be aligned with the medical center's vision (for example, the prevention program should be implicit in the budget, capital equipment purchased should relate to improving care for one of the major disease groups). Eventually, Bingham sees all departments and staff working toward the same vision of "making Magic Valley the healthiest place in America." As part of a process called "organizational visioning," each department head is expected to discuss the hospital's vision and values with staff and then discuss the alignment of his or her department's activities with the hospital's. Out of this process, each department devises its own departmental mission and quality definition. The importance of this process is expressed in a quote by Carl Jung that Fischer provided: "Without a personal vision, you can't help the organization reach its vision."

As part of their departmental rollout activities, Elizabeth Gallian, vice-president of nursing services, began investigating methods to improve nursing care. By directing and coordinating the efforts of nursing educators and the nursing management team, a philosophical practice framework was created that would support the scope and process of professional nursing. Through research efforts, Wesorick's clinical practice model[3] was identified as a vehicle congruous with Magic Valley's quality framework. This model specifically addresses variations in the current process of nursing care delivery and offers tools and resources to reduce or eliminate those variations. According to Gallian, the major objectives of Wesorick's clinical practice model are to

- delineate nursing services that flow from the scope of professional practice;
- establish a process whereby staff govern their practice and hold each other accountable for the scope and practice of professional nursing service;
- implement clinically adaptable tools/resources that support the scope and process of professional nursing practice; and
- strengthen each nurse's clarity, commitment, and valuing of professional nursing services, and the ability to educate peers, other health care providers, and consumers.

The integration of CQI into the practice of nursing at Magic Valley began with a commitment to the vision and the framework of CQI. Shared governance provides a communication structure that supports these objectives. The clinical practice model exemplifies the principles of a CQI environment.

QI Process

To approach a problem or opportunity for improvement, Magic Valley follows HCA's FOCUS-PDCA method. (See pages 34–35 of Chapter 1.) However, Quorum changed the "C" in PDCA to "S" for "study" because they believed the word "check" implies inspection. At least 20 teams are busy investigating processes across the hospital. Table 4.2 (page 116) lists some of Magic Valley's team activities, and a case study (page 117) provides the story of the breast self-exam team. Some of these teams have been formally recognized by the QIC while others have sprung up independently.

Several factors have hampered Magic Valley's team efforts, including the lack of trained facilitators, storyboards, and a full-time coach. Looking back, Bingham would have provided a course that trained facilitators early on since there have not been enough facilitators to meet the demand. The QIC also struggled for a long time with the size and style of its storyboards. While it has recently developed a format that corrected the difficulties they had with the traditional FOCUS-PDSA board (for example, difficulty in tracking), much of the initial momentum staff manifested has died down. Another barrier the organization has come across is the lack of a full-time coach. Fischer, who directs CQI training along with Linda Markt, director of education, and provides CQI consultation to staff, is also in charge of QA, infection control, and other areas. She has often had to choose between team activities and other priorities. A full-time coach "would have helped carry the momentum, provided statistical knowledge, and possibly would have arranged for more celebrations," Bingham said. Fischer cautioned organizations that do hire a full-time coach to "make sure that person is not in charge of the development of CQI in the hospital; otherwise it becomes a department function like QA," she said.

QA/QI Relationship

Staff at Magic Valley have no essential difficulties with the pairing of QA and CQI. An integrated QA/QI plan has been developed and

Table 4.2. A Sample of Magic Valley's Team Activities

Newborn/Obstetrics Team. The admission process of newborn infants is being studied with the goal of meeting the customer's needs—mothers want infants very soon after delivery. To date, collaboration has increased between physicians and nurses in obstetrics and the nursery.

Second North Team. The team is looking at the process of making patient assignments. They have identified the variation in patient needs and worker skills within the current process. Staff feel the process has improved, and assignments are more equitable.

Transport Team. This team is currently gathering data on the process for the in-house transportation of patients.

PCA Administration Team. The process of setting up a process-controlled analgesic pump with correct medications at correct rate for all patients is being investigated. The procedure was written, and the team developed an excellent training program.

Administration Team. This team, which is looking at the process of handling patient complaints in a timely manner, has successfully identified key people to call in various departments so customers now have answers quickly.

Lab Mail-In Team. The process of communication between departments to facilitate a timely lab report to the customer and proper billing of the test is being studied. The team has decreased the turnaround time for the bills and reports for the customers, and interdepartmental communication is occurring

Hematology Team. The team is investigating the process of ordering labor-intensive lab studies. Members have been successful in that differentials are only ordered on specific red blood counts rather than all, as previously performed.

Source: *Developed by Magic Valley Regional Medical Center, Twin Falls, Idaho, 1991. Reprinted with permission.*

adopted by all departments to guide their traditional QA activities (see Table 4.3, pages 124–126). Fischer views QA as one method to launch into the FOCUS-PDSA cycle. For example, Anne Erickson, director, surgical nursing, discovered a problem specific to the process for patient-controlled analgesia when evaluating all medication errors through QA and formed a team to investigate the process. Staff agree that the hospital still needs to collect data on important outcomes such as morbidity and mortality. However, as discussed on page 109, Miles emphasizes that these outcome data should be communitywide.

(continued on page 123)

Case Study
The Story of Magic Valley's Breast Self-Exam Improvement Team

Background

When a patient participates in Magic Valley's breast self-exam program, she receives a mammogram; is taught the technique of breast self-exam, including a demonstration of the breast self-exam by a registered nurse; and is educated on the importance of routine mammography in detecting early breast cancer. While the program was usually small (seven patients per clinic three afternoons a week), requests for breast self-exam appointments increased in the fall of 1990, causing a scheduling delay of 8 to 12 weeks. This increase in demand could be attributed to several factors:

- Our radiology department had recently received its accreditation only weeks after a national talk show on the subject;

- We received local news coverage about the mammography services;

- We had grant monies available to women over forty who had never received a mammogram; and

- With the approaching year end, women who had met their insurance deductible wanted their routine mammogram done when the costs would be covered by insurance.

The obvious solution would have been to increase the hours of the breast self-exam program to meet customers' expectations for timely scheduled appointments. However, that solution offered a return to status quo without improvement. What impact would increased hours have on staffing and program costs? Would the increased demand be temporary? Would an expanded program require increased clerical staff hours as well as registered nurse hours? Since adopting continuous quality improvement, we are asking more questions. How quickly do patients want routine exams scheduled? (Patients with a problem could be seen within the week.) Did other parts of our program need to be changed? Is there an opportunity for improving the program?

By forming a quality improvement team and using the FOCUS-PDSA approach, we were able to address these far-reaching issues. The following paragraphs present the steps that our team went through in investigating the breast self-exam program.

Find an opportunity. By improving the education portion of the breast self-exam process from the time a patient arrives to register until she leaves for the mammogram, staff believed they would be able to see more patients and help decrease the appointment schedule delay.

Currently, this portion of the process limits the number of patients who can be seen in an afternoon.

Organize the team. With the quality improvement focused on the education portion of the breast self-exam, it was apparent the team members needed to include

- Linda Markt, director of education and Women's Health Center, owner of this process and team leader;
- Jill Chestnut, breast self-exam practitioner and educator;
- Carol Serpa, secretary, who schedules appointments and keeps all records for the breast self-exam program;
- Betty Grant, volunteer, who registers patients when they arrive for the education/examination/mammogram;
- Jan Hyder, radiology operations manager, who performs the mammogram;
- Sharon Dingman, radiology office manager, who schedules mammogram appointments; and
- Sue Summers, director of community relations, who is the team facilitator.

Clarify current process. In this phase, we used flowcharts to define the current process and identify any time delays (see Figure 4.A, page 119). We also took the time to find what our customers thought about the program through a written questionnaire given to each patient. The questionnaire we used is provided in Figure 4.B (page 120). With this information, we identified the following improvement opportunities:

- Instead of canceling the clinic when our practitioner was unavailable, we could train a back-up nurse;
- We could simplify finding the review portion of the breast self-exam video by putting the review on a separate video; and
- We could eliminate some patient waiting by dedicating time to the clinic and not allowing other interferences.

Understand variation. Through the flowchart, we identified the following causes for delay:

- Patient arrives late;
- Patient needs help with insurance information;
- Patient does not speak English;
- Patient has difficulty completing paperwork;
- Exam room not available for patient;
- Nurse is unable to go to exam room when patient is ready;
- Patient has multiple questions and requires more exam/teaching time; and
- Patient has physical problems that require more time to move.

Figure 4.A. Breast Self-Exam Instruction Program

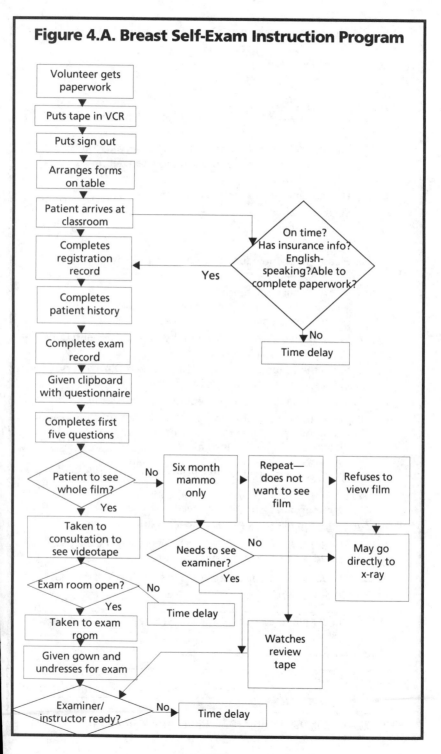

Figure 4.B. Breast Screening Program Opinionnaire

Yes No

— —   1. When you made your appointment for your breast screening and mammogram, did you receive sufficient information?

2. When scheduling a breast screening exam and mammogram, it would be acceptable to wait up to ___days
— —   or ___weeks.

— —   3. Did you appreciate the reminder call?

— —   4. Were you able to locate the Women's Health Center easily?

5. Did the volunteer greet you pleasantly and help you fill out the forms?

6. Please check the education you found helpful:

_____ movie
_____ personal teaching
_____ screening/examination
_____ pamphlets

7. What was your waiting time in the Women's Health Cen-
— —   ter?_____ Was this acceptable?

8. Were the Diagnostic Imaging Department (X-ray) personnel
— —   courteous and knowledgeable?

9. Was the mammogram procedure explained sufficiently?

10. Please indicate, if any, your level of discomfort during your mammogram (please rate from 1 to 10—that is, 1 = no discomfort, 10 = very uncomfortable):_____

11. What was your waiting time in the Diagnostic Imaging
— —   Department (X-Ray)? _____ Was it acceptable?

12. Do you think a letter telling you about your screening/
— —   mammogram results is valuable?

13. Do you plan to use the Women's Health Center Breast
— —   Screening Program for your next mammogram?

14. Would you recommend this program to your friends?

15. How did you find out about the Women's Health Center Breast Screening Program?

_____

16. What could we improve about the Breast Screening/Mammogram Program?

_____

_____

17. What did we do best?

_____

_____

Thank you for taking the time to fill out this opinionnaire.

Through the satisfaction questionnaire, we learned that patients are pleased with the breast screening exam program. The comments section included many general superlatives—"excellent," "wonderful," and "great." More specific comments told us the program was well organized, informative, giving recognition to the individual examiner, pleasant atmosphere, and so forth. However, by far the most frequent comments were about the staff. Statements included: "everyone made me feel comfortable," "everyone was helpful," "everyone was professional," and "you all smiled." Personal attention was mentioned six times. After reviewing these comments, we decided our key quality characteristic is the personal attention and sensitivity our staff demonstrate.

From the questionnaire responses, we also learned that the acceptable length of time to schedule an appointment is four weeks or less for 85% of the patients (More than 60% requested two weeks or less). The Pareto diagram in Figure 4.C (page 122) illustrates these data. Many repeat patients also informed us on the questionnaire that they would not want to see the educational video again.

Select the improvement. After evaluating the data, we decided to schedule three more patients per clinic one day per week.

Plan the improvement. Our pilot plan was to use one additional clinic per week for training another nurse. We would begin adding the three extra patients after her training was completed. To make comparisons, we anticipated that we would have to collect data for the pilot clinic and regular clinic and compare the satisfaction questionnaires from the pilot clinic with questionnaires from regular clients.

Do the pilot. After we ran six extra clinics for training, we began tracking the time for registration, video education, and self-examination instruction separately. We also kept track of the frequency of occurrence of the reasons for time delays.

Study the results. After 15 clinics, the total time for the education components was plotted on a run chart. The run chart (see Figure 4.D, page 122) shows too many runs. We interpret this to be the nature of the service, meaning we adjust the time to meet the patient's need. It also shows a range of time from 30 to 74 minutes.

Patient satisfaction responses did not change for the ten patient clinic days. The pilot study demonstrated we could schedule three more patients without creating unmanageable problems for the nurse examiner or the mammography schedule.

Act on the results. Our decision is to continue one ten-patient clinic per week. If the appointment schedule increases to three weeks, we will add three additional patients to another afternoon clinic. The true test of our team's efforts will be in the fall of 1991 when demand will increase

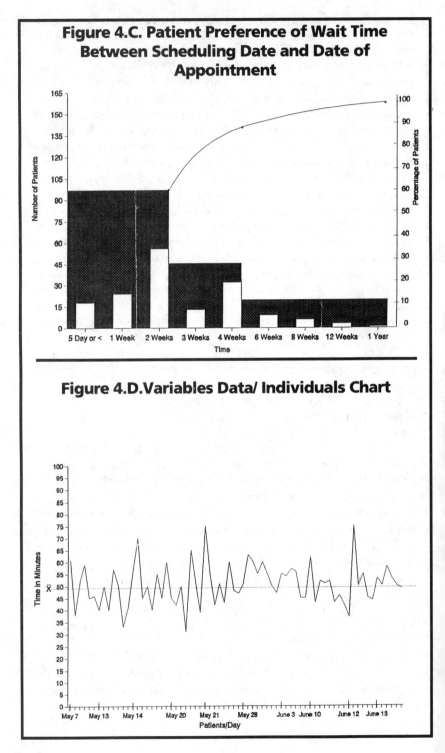

Figure 4.C. Patient Preference of Wait Time Between Scheduling Date and Date of Appointment

Figure 4.D.Variables Data/ Individuals Chart

for breast self-exams. At that time, insurance deductibles will be met and grant money will become available again.

Summary

Rather than jumping at the "obvious solution" of adding another afternoon clinic, our quality improvement effort has increased the number of breast self-exam patients seen, without adding costs. Additionally, the program has been enhanced by our efforts to improve quality. We were unaware of the patient's response to repetitive video instruction. We identified and eliminated some miscommunication about the mammogram procedure. We learned that we had allowed other programs to interfere with the registered nurse seeing breast self-exam patients and we were able to reestablish the patients as the priority. We have increased our awareness of more opportunities to improve our program. We have established a new commitment to contributing to the health of the Magic Valley community through cost-effective improvements.

Source: *Developed and written by Linda Markt, RN, director of education, Magic Valley Regional Medical Center, Twin Falls, Idaho. Reprinted with permission, 1991.*

(continued from page 116)

Education

As discussed earlier, the QIC decided to suspend training for a time until the board and senior management were anchored. CQI training is continuing from the top down at Magic Valley. Senior management, some board members, and department managers have received formal advanced courses in CQI methods and statistical thinking, and all other staff have received awareness training on the concepts of CQI as part of an annual reorientation each year. Physicians have not yet received any formal CQI training. However, to maintain staff enthusiasm and encourage process improvement, just-in-time training has been provided for all teams. Staff have also received training more indirectly as part of their departmental QI activities.

Bingham says the hospital has not yet reached the point at which it needs a statistical consultant. The hospital's board member from Universal Foods provides the hospital and other businesses in the community with many CQI resources, such as tapes of Deming lectures. Also hospital staff have attended courses sponsored by Universal.

Table 4.3. Magic Valley's Quality Assessment/ Quality Improvement (QA/QI) Plan

Magic Valley developed the following QA/QI plan to help guide departments in their QA activities and to illustrate techniques for incorporating QI concepts and tools into traditional monitoring and evaluation. For example, step VII explains that QI tools such as fishbone diagrams can be used to analyze and improve a process, and step VIII instructs staff to use the FOCUS-PDCA framework for improvement purposes

I. **Purpose**
    To provide a guide to identify, coordinate, and plan and pursue opportunities to continually improve the quality of health care and services we provide. We understand that patients as well as staff members may have different values, cultural beliefs, perceptions, and expectations of health, illness, health care, and quality of life that can affect patient/staff interactions, the quality of patient care and services, and clinical outcomes.

II. **Responsibility**
    The department manager, under the direction of _____, is responsible for QA/QI activities. The_____, or his/her designee, shall report status and results of QA/QI/risk management activities, with recommendations to be reported to the hospitalwide QA/QI Committee.

III. **Scope of care**
    The _____ department provides _____ diagnostic exams and/or therapeutic procedures from_____ AM to_____PM at_____for inpatients and/or outpatients (circle as applicable). These services are provided by

    _____.

IV. **Important aspects of care**
    Those aspects of care and services that occur frequently, affect large numbers of patients, place the patient at risk, or tend to produce problems for patients or staff are selected for QA/QI.

V. **Monitoring indicators—criteria for evaluation**
    The monitoring indicators are developed and reviewed annually. They are based on high-risk, high-volume, and/or problem-prone areas. An indicator may be identified as a result of FOCUS. The results of monitoring activities are summarized and reported according to the QA calendar. Monitoring indicators are selected, developed, and/or adapted

Table 4.3. Magic Valley's Quality Assessment/ Quality Improvement (QA/QI) Plan (continued)

by staff members and approved by the department. Indicators are of two general types, sentinel event and rate based. Events indicators may measure are outcomes, processes, desirable outcomes, and undesirable outcomes. Preestablished criteria are used to evaluate the indicators/monitors for compliance with department and hospital policies and procedures.

VI. **Collect and organize data**
Existing sources of potentially useful data sources are patient records, department logs, committee meeting minutes or reports, infection control reports, patient questionnaires, observation of patients or staff, and utilization review findings. To collect and organize data, the following must be determined for each indicator:
1. The data source;
2. The data collection method
3. The appropriateness of sampling; and
4. The frequency of data collection.

VII. **Analyze data**
Data are regularly analyzed as part of the QI activity. Specific opportunities for improvement are identified. Techniques that assist in understanding the contributory processes in a system (for example, fishbone diagrams), the connections among processes (for example, flowcharts), and the relative contributions to process variation (for example, Pareto charts) are used to analyze the process and identify methods to reduce variation and improve performance.

VIII. **Actions to solve identified problems/opportunities for improvement**
If the evaluation process identifies a problem or an opportunity for improvement, the staff decide what corrective action is necessary. When possible, the FOCUS-PDCA framework and tools will be used for continuous process improvement.
The effectiveness of any actions taken are assessed and documented. Continuous process improvement is encouraged. Therefore, when actions are necessary to solve problems, they are taken and the effectiveness of the action(s) taken is assessed.
Sources of variation are sought within organizational processes, rather than individuals. Recommended actions to improve the quality of the process of patient care and services will be put into effect to eliminate, or to appropriately

Table 4.3. Magic Valley's Quality Assessment/ Quality Improvement (QA/QI) Plan (continued)

reduce, identified variations. These actions may include
1. orientation;
2. continuing education;
3. preceptorship; and
4. informative management.

IX. **Communication**
Monitoring and evaluation, including findings, conclusions, and recommendations, is communicated to the organizationwide QA/ QI program formally on a quarterly basis. In addition, open and less formal communication occurs between department managers, the Quality Resources Director, or other hospital personnel during the entire QI process. A storyboard could facilitate this communication.

X. **QA/QI calendar**

XI. **QA/QI forms**

XII. **Annual evaluation**
The program is to be reviewed annually by the department of _____. A summary of the evaluation will be reported to the hospitalwide QA/QI Committee.

XIII. **Review and approval**

Source: Developed by Magic Valley Regional Medical Center, Twin Falls, Idaho, 1990. Reprinted with permission.

Bingham considers the fact that senior managers and department managers become trainers themselves key to the success of their education effort. "If an organization is not a teaching organization," Bingham said, "it won't get there." Quorum has encouraged self-sufficiency in all the organizations it manages rather than a dependency on consultants. While Magic Valley brought Quorum in to help senior managers learn CQI methods and tools, the hospital plans to "become self-sufficient internally," Bingham said. The QI coach and others in the QIC are developing their own curriculum, and senior management have been leading the courses.

Since Magic Valley's efforts extend beyond the hospital, the QIC and board have begun to help arrange for members of the community to receive CQI training. The board is working diligently to persuade the local junior college to offer courses on CQI to the community.

QI Supports

As part of the infrastructure senior management are building to support the CQI rollout, they considered several practical issues, such as providing process-related data to teams and reward and recognition to staff. The following are several support efforts that are assisting the hospital move toward CQI.

Customer feedback mechanisms. Recent monthly focus groups have assisted the board in formulating the hospital's direction. According to Sue Summers, public relations/marketing director, the hospital randomly invites people in the community to the focus groups. Each group focuses on the vision of the hospital and asks attendees to identify their number one concern about health care. The same three concerns have ranked high at each focus group: need for more physicians, emphasis on education and preventive health, and affordable care. After considering this information, the board is diligently recruiting more physicians and putting more emphasis on preventive health. Summers believes the participants in the focus groups "tell you things they wouldn't tell you on a questionnaire" and tells how one participant said the group helped "water the wallflowers," or encourage people to participate. However, Summers stresses the need to mix the forms of customer data. In addition to the focus groups, external customer information is gained through Quorum's hospital quality trend survey, which allows Magic Valley to compare its services to those of other hospitals managed by Quorum; department-level surveys; and informal interviews of patients at their bedsides.

Information system. Magic Valley is in the process of installing a new wide-area network computer system. Making extensive use of personal computers at work stations throughout the hospital, the system will allow access to existing, previously independent systems serving the laboratory and radiology services. Patient data base information and clinical information will also be available to appropriate users of the system in the hospital, and data studies can be developed from any point in the hospital. Easy access to all patient data bases and the hospital's administrative data bases will facilitate the availability of data to teams. In addition, new data needs will be more flexibly met as teams and their projects develop in the future. Tests of the system have been successful to date. Final implementation is anticipated in December 1991.

Shared compensation. Magic Valley eliminated its merit pay system about two years ago and substituted a shared compensation program, which links employee increases to the financial health of the hospital. Staff still receive annual performance evaluations without rankings, but the evaluations do not affect compensation. "Adopting the Deming philosophy helped us realize we had to do something different. The old way was effective, but fear was involved. You unhook the money and you unhook the fear," said Rosemary Barta, human resources director. Before undertaking the new sharing system, Magic Valley hired an outside company to help them align employee salaries with the market and reduce the variation among salaries within the hospital. Each job description was analyzed and a fair salary attached. Then to ensure that all employees receive a cost-of-living compensation, the hospital provided for a 3% increase for all employees each year. Any additional salary adjustment, however, is determined through the sharing program and depends on the hospital's financial bottom line. The amount available is based on a portion of the salary budget. For example, $300,000 was available last year. If the hospital remains in budget, the $300,000 is divided among employees. Shares differ according to the hours employees work (that is, full-time, part-time). Most staff receive a 2% to 4% raise through the sharing program; this is in addition to the 3% annual increase.

Magic Valley's new compensation system ties each employee to the hospital's successes and failures. Rewards are based on group performance, not job title or percent of base pay. "We were amazed how little staff knew about financial management of the organization," Bingham said. While Bingham acknowledged that Magic Valley has a long way go in developing an appropriate compensation system, he said that "staff have started becoming interested in why they sometimes get a share and other times don't."

One issue Barta hopes to address in the near future is how to reward the excellent performer. This issue was not addressed by the merit system, which was too subjective and tended to benefit the average performer, Barta explained. The response of many staff within the merit system was "I stand on my head and still get an average raise," she said. Although Magic Valley has some programs in place, such as the "moment of truth" program, in which patients and staff can nominate a staff person for doing something special for a patient, Barta is looking into a more substantive reward mechanism.

Supplier relationships. Magic Valley is also using CQI principles in its relationships with suppliers. For example, the hospital brainstormed a list of problems with a cross-functional group related to problems with Baxter's intravenous products. Baxter Healthcare sent two people from Chicago to work out the time lines on necessary changes related to back orders, breakage, and so forth. (Magic Valley's QI efforts with suppliers are aided in part by their relationship with Quorum, which contracts with many suppliers for all the hospitals it manages. Quorum has set up formal agreements with these companies asking that they participate in QI endeavors.)

Physician Involvement

The QIC decided up front to wait to involve physicians in CQI activities. One reason the QIC hesitated to involve physicians was the fear that they would have difficulty providing the proper resources (for example, facilitators, data) needed to carry out CQI once physicians became intrigued. Magic Valley decided to enlist physician support indirectly at first. In a unique move, Bingham encouraged Miles to implement CQI techniques in his office, hoping physicians would become excited by the results. Bingham felt this may be a more "marketable" approach than attacking internal processes head-on. Staff at Magic Valley point out several other approaches hospitals might use to enlist physicians in CQI: involve hospital-based physicians (for example, pathologists) who show an interest in learning about CQI, seek physician's input when addressing processes that affect them, and invite an expert on CQI in clinical areas to speak to the medical staff. Looking back, Bingham feels it may have been better to involve physicians earlier in their CQI effort.

Conclusion

Adopting the concepts of CQI has made staff and board members at Magic Valley look beyond the walls of the medical center. Replacing the competitive methods many hospitals took up during the 1980s, Magic Valley is embracing cooperativeness and community involvement. With the concepts of systems thinking in mind, staff recognized that the diagnosis and treatment of patients, which occurs within the walls of the medical center, is only one part of the larger health care system that begins with education and prevention. Signs are appearing that Magic Valley's efforts to spread CQI understanding through the community are beginning to pay off. The president-elect of the Chamber of Commerce has pledged that he would use CQI methods at the Chamber, and several churches in town have begun using CQI methods. There is also talk in town of beginning a communitywide QIC. "To the extent that these agencies [other businesses, city government] start understanding CQI, ...it will help us leverage a cultural transformation of the community," Bingham said. The activities being pursued at Magic Valley raise some exciting questions about the paradigm shift occurring within hospitals moving toward CQI.

References

1. Senge PM: *The Fifth Discipline.* New York: Doubleday/Currency, 1990.

2. Bronowski J: *Science and Human Values.* New York: Harper & Row, Publishers, Inc, 1965.

3. Wesorick B: *Standards of Nursing Care: A Model for Clinical Practice.* Philadelphia: JB Lippincott, 1990.

5 Building a House of Quality
Bethesda Hospital, Inc
Cincinnati, Ohio

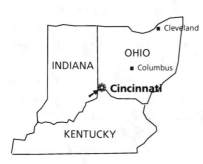

Type of hospital: Not-for-profit community hospital

Scope of service: General medical/surgical

Beds: 701, with an average census of 502, between two hospitals—Bethesda North and Bethesda Oak

Extent of involvement in TQM: Since 1988, Bethesda has been using Hoshin planning and quality function deployment to guide their rollout of TQM. Over 40 teams are investigating both administrative and clinical processes, including a team that is working with an outside supplier.

Special aspects of TQM:
— GOAL/QPC approach that involves Hoshin planning, cross-functional management, and daily management
— Antecedent environment that emphasized data-based innovation
— Extending TQM to supplier relationships
— Information system that supports TQM
— Application of breakthrough thinking
— Hybrid 13-step problem-solving method
— Strong customer-supplier tracking system, including use of quality function deployment
— Criteria established for measuring success
— Early involvement of medical staff

The foundation of Bethesda's total quality management (TQM) initiative was laid about 20 years ago when L. Thomas Wilburn, Jr, arrived at the hospital as vice-president and manager of the Oak Street Hospital. Wilburn came to Bethesda from Community Hospital of Indiana, Inc where he had established one of the first hospital system engineering departments and experimented with applying statistical process control across many hospital functions. Surrounding himself with creative and innovative staff, Wilburn began exploring new ventures. Bethesda has been among the first hospitals to try new procedures (for example, microvascular free tissue flap, fetal monitoring), acquire revolutionary equipment (for example, MRI technology), and begin new programs (for example, free-standing outpatient surgery center in 1977, Bethesda-managed employee fitness centers). But never far from the ideas at Bethesda are the data to back them up. "Innovation is a synthesis of what you see around you," says Will Groneman, chief operating officer of Bethesda Oak. "You see something you think is worthwhile, then gather data to see if the idea was a good idea . . . quantification allows us to implement what we do as well as we do." The culture that Wilburn began constructing back in the 1970s served as a springboard to TQM. The hospital's approach to TQM reflects the dual emphasis on data and creative breakthrough inherent at Bethesda. Bethesda is piloting a ten-element implementation strategy[1] developed by GOAL/QPC, a consulting firm in Methuen, Massachusetts, and using Japanese quality improvement methods such as Hoshin planning, daily management, and cross-functional management, which includes quality function deployment (QFD).

The GOAL/QPC approach has helped staff understand "the multiple confluences of TQM," said Sue Weinstein, MD, medical staff consultant. Teams are actively investigating dozens of processes, both administrative and clinically related. But far from restricting TQM to team activities, staff are beginning to use TQM on a daily basis to improve processes in their own departments, and both hospitals are focused on increasing timeliness of all services through Hoshin planning. Involving staff in more aspects of TQM than teamwork has begun to create a climate where day-to-day activities are carried out in the "context of quality," says Jim Connelly, chief operating officer, Bethesda North. TQM has given Mary Beth Durnell, manager, social services, "an opportunity to think differently . . . . Even in a crisis, I am looking at the cause, doing a mini cause-and-effect diagram in my mind." Durnell says. "Now I tend to think in terms of breaking down barriers, collaboration, how is this going to affect so and so." As a result, she feels department walls are becoming "more permeable."

Description and Demographics

The Cincinnati skyline resembles a collage of Fortune 500 companies. Lining the Ohio River are such names as Procter & Gamble, Chiquita Brands, Kroger, EW Scripps, American Financial, Charter, Federated, and Allied Stores. Connelly suggests that Bethesda's data-based innovation resembles the methods these companies have found profitable. "Cincinnati is a town known for its conservatism," he says, "yet when you step back and look at the success of the companies represented here, all are strong risk takers but in a deliberate way." Cincinnati's start as a major business center began with the opening of the Miami Canal. Named the "Queen City of the West" by Henry Wadsworth Longfellow, Cincinnati became a stopping ground for settlers on their way west. Many stayed on including large numbers of German immigrants who gave the city its rich European heritage. While people have long stopped traveling by river boat, more than 46 million tons of cargo still pass through the Port of Cincinnati each year.

The fourteenth largest employer in Cincinnati, Bethesda, Inc, is a private, not-for-profit, diversified health care organization made up of

- two acute care hospitals;
- a home health agency;
- a durable medical equipment company;
- a senior services division, which operates two nursing facilities and an adult day care center; and
- Bethesda Healthcare, Inc, which includes the operation of two work capacity centers; five occupational health centers; and numerous contractual services provided to medium-size and large-size businesses, including employee assistance programs, occupational health nursing services, and management contracts for the operation of corporate fitness centers for 12 major industries in Cincinnati.

Bethesda Oak is the urban hospital with 434 beds, and Bethesda North is the suburban hospital with 333 beds. With a combined medical staff of over 1,300, the two hospitals are able to offer a broad spectrum of outpatient and inpatient services including alcohol/chemical dependency, cardiac rehabilitation, cardiac catheterization, CT, infertility, intensive care, laser surgery, lithotripsy, MRI, neonatal intensive care, oncology services, outpatient surgery, rehabilitation outpatient services, sleep disorders center, and sports medicine. Approximately 29,000 are admitted to Bethesda each year; patients are drawn from a young middle class population (the median age in the Cincinnati area is 32.4 years). Fifty-six percent of the hospital's gross patient revenue is derived from Medicare and Medicaid.

History

Although Bethesda has been using industrial management techniques for almost two decades, the hospital did not make a commitment to TQM until the late 1980s. "If the organization is not ready [to move to TQM]", Wilburn said, "it won't fly." He began to "plant the seeds" at first, talking about TQM and Deming, bringing in external speakers, and showing videos to senior management "to get the language accepted." In 1988, senior management attended the four-day seminar presented by Dr Edwards Deming where they became convinced that TQM "made sense," Wilburn said.

Key to Bethesda's TQM effort was the selection of GOAL/QPC as its consultant. In the summer of 1988, Wilburn attended the National Demonstration Project Conference where he heard the 21 hospitals involved report on their activities. Impressed by the approach GOAL/QPC had taken when working with one of the hospitals, Wilburn sought out Bob King, executive director of GOAL/QPC. The firm had a substantial record of research and activity with major manufacturing industries. At first, Wilburn had difficulty recruiting GOAL/QPC. Eventually, however, the hospital set up a consulting arrangement with the firm. Bethesda is the first hospital with which the firm has worked comprehensively. It is also the alpha site for GOAL/QPC's new ten-element implementation model (see Figure 5.1, page 135). The hospital's TQM story has progressed along the ten steps in GOAL/QPC's original implementation plan. While working at Bethesda, GOAL/QPC has been able to further develop the model.

Top group decides to do TQM. After Wilburn returned from the National Demonstration Project Meeting, he and senior management agreed to make an organizationwide commitment to TQM and began setting their efforts in full swing. A Steering Committee, which included all senior management and several medical staff leaders, was formed in January 1989 to lead the effort. About the same time, two staff persons were hired, giving Bethesda "the cadre of talent they needed to begin implementing and pushing TQM out in the organi-

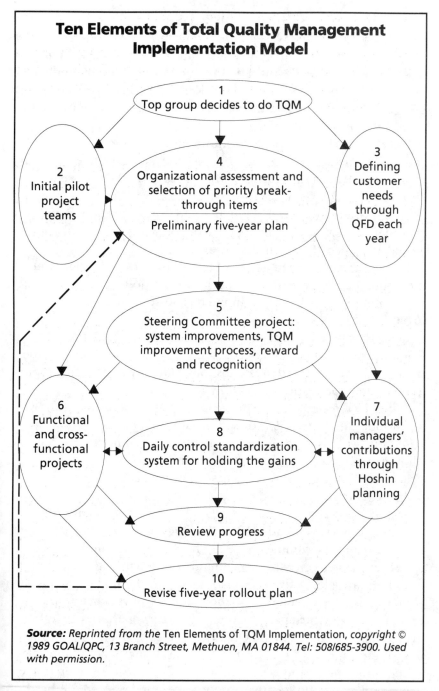

Ten Elements of Total Quality Management Implementation Model

1 Top group decides to do TQM

2 Initial pilot project teams

4 Organizational assessment and selection of priority break-through items

Preliminary five-year plan

3 Defining customer needs through QFD each year

5 Steering Committee project: system improvements, TQM improvement process, reward and recognition

6 Functional and cross-functional projects

8 Daily control standardization system for holding the gains

7 Individual managers' contributions through Hoshin planning

9 Review progress

10 Revise five-year rollout plan

Source: Reprinted from the Ten Elements of TQM Implementation, copyright © 1989 GOAL/QPC, 13 Branch Street, Methuen, MA 01844. Tel: 508/685-3900. Used with permission.

Figure 5.1. Bethesda is the alpha site for GOAL-QPC's ten-step implementation model.

zation," Wilburn says. Hired in 1988 as director of corporate education, Gerry Kaminski was asked to become the vice-president of TQM as well. "We realized education was so much a part of TQM," Wilburn said, "it seemed like a natural tie to put education and management of TQM together as responsibilities." Kaminski also had the benefit of bringing both clinical and managerial health care experience to her new role (see "Education").

From his early attempts to institute industrial methods in health care, Wilburn felt it was crucial to involve the medical staff early on. As soon as Sue Weinstein's resume crossed his desk, Wilburn sent her a copy of Deming's *Out of the Crisis*. A physician with an MBA from the Wharton Graduate School of Finance and Administration, Weinstein agreed to undertake the challenge of introducing TQM to physicians at Bethesda (see "Physician Involvement").

Bethesda was fortunate to have a board that backed their commitment to TQM from the start and appropriated dollars toward it; many board members work for Cincinnati businesses that are also involved in TQM.

Once they had the structure in place to roll out TQM, the Steering Committee identified the concepts of TQM they found most important, which are discussed in "Philosophy." Quality 1 was then adopted as the theme for Bethesda's TQM effort.

Initial pilot project teams. The hospital began experimenting with TQM tools and methods. Advised by GOAL/QPC to select projects based on "what is causing pain," the Steering Committee set up six pilot teams in the spring of 1989 to analyze a cross-corporate mix of processes. These pilots were successful primarily for the lessons and insights gained.

Defining customer needs through QFD. An advanced TQM tool, QFD exercises assist staff in statistically analyzing and prioritizing customer needs. During the summer of 1989, the Steering Committee piloted a QFD exercise to give them a general knowledge of the tool and to help them develop a five-year plan. First they defined the hospital's primary customers: patients and their families, physicians, employers, employees, and third-party payers. Then they gathered together a group of physicians from the Quality 1 medical staff advisory group to determine what was important to them and what made them select Bethesda as a preferred place to practice. The physicians then ranked each item based on relative importance and assessed Bethesda's position as compared to its competitors.

Selection of breakthrough objectives and development of five-year plan. Based on feedback from the first six pilot teams and the QFD exercise, the Steering Committee identified three breakthrough objectives that prioritized the organization's TQM efforts:

• Identify and improve customer/supplier relationships;

• Enhance Bethesda's position as the preferred place to work and the preferred place for physicians to practice; and

• Improve accuracy and timeliness of services and maintain these gains.

With these three objectives in mind, the Steering Committee developed a task-oriented five-year plan, which defines a comprehensive list of tasks to take Bethesda through 1993 (see "Strategy").

Steering Committee projects. Coincident with other TQM activities, Bethesda's Steering Committee began several formal and informal projects to investigate systemwide processes that affect the roll out of TQM, including the operating budget system, review and improvement of the TQM process, and reward and recognition of teams and individuals. In addition, three cross-functional management teams were formed to address organizational transformation, making Bethesda the preferred place to work, and holding the gains. The organizational transformation team began by discussing and debating the meaning and application of Deming's 14 points. They progressed to envisioning new management behaviors within a TQM organization. Those behaviors the team felt management should "walk" within a TQM hospital are listed in Table 5.1 (page 138). "We're trying to get managers to 'do' good rather than 'act' good," says Tom Maggart, senior vice-president and chief financial officer. "The culture of the past was trying to reward people who look good. This did not encourage risk taking and was the cause of considerable finger pointing."

Midway into 1991, Bethesda is making progress along steps 6, 7, and 8 of the implementation plan. As discussed further in "QI Process" and "Strategy," more than 40 teams are investigating a variety of functional and cross-functional processes, and Hoshin planning and daily management are being piloted in several areas of the organization.

Philosophy

Early in their TQM initiative, the Steering Committee approved a statement of purpose: "To adopt a leadership philosophy that supports, encourages, and expects all employees to participate in the

e 5.1. Management Behaviors Within a TQM Organization

Consider the priorities of the organization when making decisions

Define staff expectations, roles, and responsibilities clearly

- Lead employees toward process improvement, customer orientation, and team orientation—provide framework for things to change/improve

- Facilitate a process for developing solutions

- Require data-based or information-based decision making

- Allow subordinates to make less-than-optimal solutions and then discuss with them ways to improve decision making

- Think through all functions needed and involve them before decision is made

- Recognize the difference between special and common causes

- Build consensus

- Behave as coaches, not bosses

- Encourage the sharing of successes/problems so all can learn

Source: Reprinted with permission from Bethesda Hospital, Inc, Cincinnati, Ohio, 1991.

continuous improvement of services to meet the health care needs of the community." The Steering Committee drew on the concepts and teachings of Deming when developing the philosophical structure to support its TQM effort. His influence is seen in the Quality 1 core concepts they developed: focus on the customer, reduction in variation, continuous improvement, and teamwork.

Bethesda's strategy is based on the belief that it is more valuable for the entire organization to concentrate on improving a few key areas (that is, Hoshin planning) than to have teams move in different, often conflicting directions. Kaminski stresses that while ideally staff at Bethesda are empowered, they "should be empowered in a specific direction." One of Bethesda's TQM goals is "to support and recognize departmental and cross-functional teamwork." Wilburn says this goal recognizes "that the things that benefit a department may not benefit an organization." Bethesda has involved staff in quality planning from the very beginning of the Quality 1 initiative "so they would recognize the impact of their actions on others," Wilburn said. Bethesda "learned early on that teams were not the whole process," Kaminski said. GOAL/QPC's approach showed staff the big picture from the beginning, "rather than allowing us to have 45 teams going and two years later not understanding how they fit into the larger structure." she said.

Bethesda is also incorporating the breakthrough thinking ideas of Gerald Nadler,[2] a professor at the University of Southern California (USC), who emphasizes there is "nothing so useless as doing something perfect that doesn't need to be done," Wilburn said. Wilburn was introduced to Nadler's thinking when he took a sabbatical in 1962 at USC to study work design. Nadler's use of the word *breakthrough* is different from the Hoshin concept of breakthrough objectives. Nadler's breakthrough thinking is "an approach to planning, design, and problem solving that translates ideas into actions." As discussed further in "QI Process," Bethesda has incorporated some of Nadler's principles into its 13-step process improvement model and has begun piloting teams that approach projects using Nadler's principles.

Strategy

"Planning" does not begin to describe Bethesda's comprehensive, top-to-bottom, horizontally integrated strategy illustrated by the GOAL/QPC wheel in Figure 5.2 (page 140). Bethesda's strategy involves staff across the organization in identifying and achieving breakthrough objectives that will exceed customer expectations. As the wheel shows, this integration occurs in three directions:

- Vertically staff use *Hoshin planning* to maximize focus on strategic targets from the chief executive officer to line employees;
- Within each department or unit, staff are involved in *daily management* to maximize department and individual performance every day; and
- Horizontally staff use *cross-functional management*, which includes QFD, to maximize coordination and cooperation among all related functions.

Bethesda is still piloting all these elements in different areas of the organization. When their strategy is fully integrated, it will be led by a customer-driven master plan. The Steering Committee will gather information from the three elements to determine strategy and then disseminate information to drive improvement activities across the organization. The following provides more details on the three components of the wheel.

Hoshin planning. In its simplest terms, Hoshin planning[3] is a game of "catch ball" between management and staff. Management begins by

139

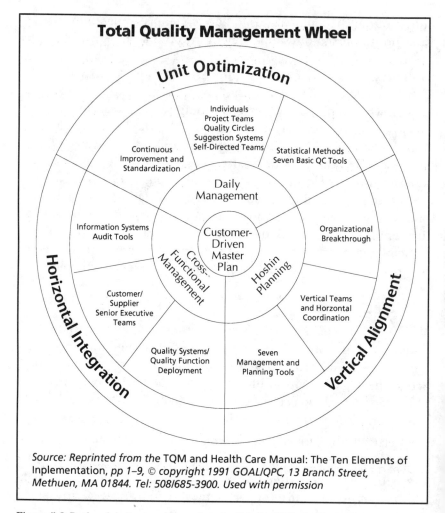

Figure 5.2. Bethesda's strategy is based on the GOAL-QPC wheel, which is divided into three sections: unit optimization, vertical alignment, and horizontal integration.

identifying a vision and breakthrough objectives that will allow the organization to achieve the vision. As shown in Figure 5.3 (page 141) top management then passes these priorities down through the levels of the organization to determine the feasibility and practicality of the objectives. Department managers in turn share their views on how they can achieve the breakthrough objectives in their specific areas. The point of Hoshin is to build consensus and vertical alignment among staff. Integral to this process is the use of the seven management and planning tools such as the affinity diagram, interrelationship diagraph, and tree diagram (see Appendix A, page 255).[4] While only management-level staff are trained in Hoshin strategy, line staff become involved in improving the processes identified through the Hoshin planning process.

Bethesda began piloting Hoshin planning in three major business segments in 1990: Bethesda Oak Hospital, Bethesda North Hospital, and corporate services. Of the three breakthrough areas the Steering Committee identified, the hospital decided to concentrate first on improving timeliness by reducing the number of customer delays. For example, the results reporting team found variation in the time it took to return reports to physician offices. Staff discovered that many reports were being mailed after the daily mail pickup, resulting in

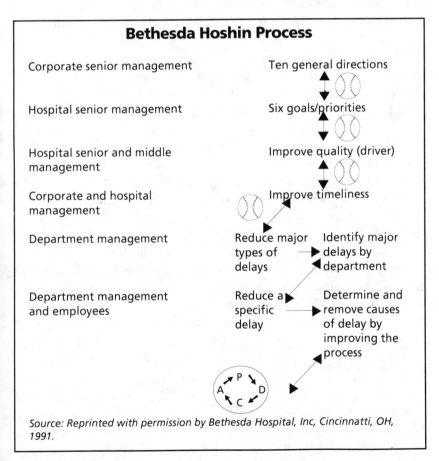

Bethesda Hoshin Process

Corporate senior management	Ten general directions
Hospital senior management	Six goals/priorities
Hospital senior and middle management	Improve quality (driver)
Corporate and hospital management	Improve timeliness
Department management	Reduce major types of delays → Identify major delays by department
Department management and employees	Reduce a specific delay → Determine and remove causes of delay by improving the process

Source: Reprinted with permission by Bethesda Hospital, Inc, Cincinnatti, OH, 1991.

Figure 5.3. Hoshin Planning is compared to a game of catch ball in this figure, where priorities are passed back and forth between the levels of an organization to determine the feasibility and practicality of the objectives.

delays. Social work discovered a different situation when investigating social workers' on-call response. Data indicated that social workers were responding in a timely fashion when paged. Social workers are now showing the data to their customers to determine what their definition of "on call" is and to try to change their perception that social workers are late in responding. Kaminski says they are refining Hoshin as they go along. She anticipates that by 1992 they will have a clearer understanding of what Hoshin can do at Bethesda.

Daily management.[5] Departments are using problem-solving techniques to improve the critical processes within their spheres as well as looking at timeliness issues through Hoshin planning. In the three business units where Bethesda has begun piloting daily management, staff determined their key customers (both internal and external), the processes that are important to their customers, and how to measure those processes. The seven quality control tools (for example, flowcharts, control charts discussed in Appendix A) are key in daily management.[6] Through this process, departments began seeing that "there are probably processes or parts of processes that are not value added," Kaminski says. "The question is, 'Do they have to be done?'" Eventually, perhaps as early as 1992, Kaminski foresees Hoshin planning linked closely with daily management activities.

Cross-functional management. In addition to aligning the organization vertically, Bethesda is ensuring that departments and divisions are working toward common goals. Key to achieving this cross-functional focus is using the voice of the customer as a guide for strategic activity. Bethesda aims not only to meet customer needs but to exceed them through QFD.[7] After the Steering Committee identified the organization's five key customers, it delegated responsibility for facilitating QFD analyses and tracking customer expectations to the marketing department. An advanced tool (only a handful of staff at Bethesda are, or will ever have to be, trained in its use), QFD analyses can be performed to identify customer needs on the entire organization (macrolevel) or concerning specific departments or programs (microlevel).

When performing QFD analyses, marketing follows the eight steps that make up the "house of quality," which is described in Figure 5.4 (page 143). Reduced to its simplest parts, the QFD team determines *what* customers want and then statistically arrives at the best methods (that is, *how*) for predicting that the customer's wants will be satisfied. By the time the QFD team completes the house of quality, they have

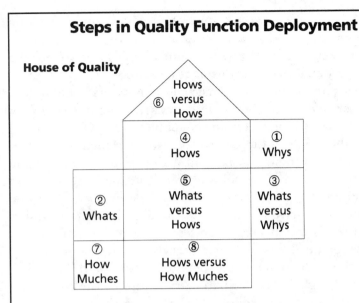

Steps in Quality Function Deployment

House of Quality

Developing the House of Quality

1. Whys: Defines the customers and competitors in the market
2. Whats: Defines customers needs and wants (spoken customer requirements)
3. Whats versus Whys: Prioritizes customer wants and identifies customer perceptions of how well you and competitors are performing on meetings their needs
4. Hows: Identifies the controllable "hows" for predicting customer satisfaction
5. Whats versus Hows: Defines relationships between Whats and Hows and priortizes the Hows
6. Hows versus Hows: Synergy/conflicts between the Hows
7. How Muches:Direction of improvements. Target values, importance of Hows
8. Hows versus How Muches: Actual calculations to determine which How will best meet a specific customer requirement

Source: *Reprinted with permission from the International Technegroup Incorporated (ITT), Milford, OH.*

Figure 5.4. When performing QFD exercises, Bethesda follows the eight steps that make up the House of Quality.

evaluated and prioritized all possible relationships and conflicts involved in providing the service or product to the customer. For example, marketing is currently facilitating a QFD analysis for the North Hospital emergency department by asking a group of emergency squad paramedics and physicians (customers) about their needs and wants concerning the emergency department (the *whats* in the house of quality). Once this step is completed, the QFD team will brainstorm the *hows*, or the controllable measurements to put in place, to predict customer satisfaction. With the help of an intricate software package, the relationships between the *whats*, the *hows*, and the *how muches* are statistically determined. "After completing the house of quality, we have a better understanding of the prioritization of customer needs and specific processes that need to be improved to meet customer needs," says Janet Stacey, manager of marketing services. Bethesda has completed about a half dozen QFDs to date. GOAL/QPC "taught us the evolutionary nature of the structure," Kaminski said. "You never just do one QFD . . . .[We] are going to have to redo them again and again."

The five-year plan. Bethesda has a five-year plan to guide them through the wheel. The plan is broken down by the tasks to be performed each year in 12 areas, including Hoshin planning, organizational transformation, Steering Committee, and customer focus. Each year, the Steering Committee reviews the progress they have made, identifies the remaining problems, and revises their five-year plan accordingly. An annual plan is then created to guide them through each year. Part of this five-year plan is the development of critical measures. The Steering Committee decided up front that increasing quality as opposed to decreasing costs should be the focus of their TQM efforts. While management sees cost reduction as a legitimate goal in the future, the ten measures currently approved by the Steering Committee are

- quality of nursing care index;
- mortality—perioperative and by service;
- nosocomial infections;
- quality deviation indicators by severity;
- average results reporting time by department;
- customer satisfaction including physicians, employers, patients, third-party payers, and persons on the street;
- employee satisfaction;

- employer preference;
- inpatient admissions market share; and
- number of admissions.

Bethesda used TQM methods to arrive at the ten measures. Staff determined the criteria they felt important for selecting a measure, such as each measure should be critical to long-term viability, focused on efficiency and timeliness, and related to the corporate vision. After brainstorming possible measures, staff used a matrix tool (see Appendix A, page 255) to narrow the list down to the ten measures listed in the preceding paragraph.

Bethesda is just beginning to gather data on these measures, Groneman said. Some of the data are available from traditional QA (that is, nosocomial infections), but staff are developing new systems to gather information on others (for example, results reporting time by department). Groneman views these measures "as preliminary. If you think of them as permanent, it can lead to paralysis," he says. For example, he hopes to develop more process-related measures in the future since the ten current measures primarily focus on outcomes.

QI Process

"There are some elements that the [GOAL/QPC] wheel doesn't give a sense of," Kaminski said. "One is that teams and education are mixed throughout and another is that the wheel is a vehicle for organizational transformation." Besides the Quality 1 teams that the Steering Committee charters, teams are popping up in departments and across disciplines to explore issues uncovered through Hoshin planning and daily management. All these teams use the same 13-step process improvement model that Bethesda developed after exploring other problem-solving approaches. Table 5.2 (page 146) illustrates the 13-step approach, and a case study (page 148) illustrates how the patient availability team used this approach. This model differs from the Shewhart cycle in that several of the steps incorporate Nadler's breakthrough thinking.[2] Step 1 instructs the team to "identify the purpose of the process," which correlates with Nadler's purposes principle. By first asking what need the organization has for a particular process, teams may avoid working on the wrong problem. Step 6 (decide what data to collect) incorporates Nadler's belief that the information collected should be limited. Teams at Bethesda determine what data will provide them with the information they are

Table 5.2. Bethesda's Process Improvement Model

1. Identify the purpose of the process
2. Identify and meet with key people
3. Describe the process
4. Define process improvement
5. Explore causes
6. Decide what data to collect
7. Collect data
8. Analyze data and identify root causes
9. Determine the action(s) to be taken
10. Create an action plan
11. Implement and pilot test the action plan
12. Evaluate the results
13. Plan for continuous improvement

Source: *Reprinted with permission from Bethesda Hospital, Inc, Cincinnati, Ohio, 1991.*

seeking rather than randomly collecting data. This step helps avoid the problem of becoming "data rich, information poor," Kaminski says, a situation she terms DRIP.

Three types of Quality 1 teams are improving processes within Bethesda: cross-functional teams, mini teams, and department teams.

Cross-functional teams. About three times a year, the Steering Committee reviews and approves formal teams to investigate processes for improvement. Each group of teams is called a round. Approximately three rounds of teams begin each year. By Fall 1991, the hospital began its sixth round of teams. Table 5.3 (page 147) provides a list of many of the teams operating at Bethesda. Projects are selected from across the organization with the three breakthrough areas in mind. Eventually, Hoshin planning, QFD, and daily process management will drive this selection process. An important enhancement to the project selection process has been the addition of a specific project clarification session that brings together the team sponsor, leader, facilitator, key management, and physicians in the area to narrow and define the charge to the team and to assemble information about the current situation, including identifying the "quality characteristics," which can be measured and expected to change as a result of the product.

(continued on page 154)

Table 5.3. A Sample of Bethesda's Quality 1 Team Activities

Completed Teams

Outpatient Billing Team. The team reduced, by approximately 48%, the time required in processing the billing of accounts for patients who registered without insurance information.

Laundry Services to Nurseries Team. The team reduced laundry product costs by $10,792 annually by reviewing and changing products and improving deliveries of clean laundry to units so that 96% of linen is delivered at or before 9:00 am.

Senior Services Nurse Aide Retention Team. The team's work contributed to the increased average length of stay of a nurse aide at Bethesda's two nursing facilities—Montgomery Care by 100% and at Scarlet Oaks by 27%.

Managed Care in Emergency Department Team. The team created a managed care provider pathway in management information systems, which identifies providers by specialty and their associated managed care plan. This pathway resulted in a 22.4% decrease in mismatches between the specialty physician called and the patient's insurance coverage.

Corporate Health Team. The team investigated how to improve the process by which patients are referred to and between various Bethesda facilities and services to ensure continuity of care for Corporate Health clients and their employees. It was able to increase client satisfaction by 73%.

Active Teams

Wound Closure Product Team. The team is approaching ways to improve the process of ordering, receiving, and paying and reordering of suture products. Suppliers are involved on this team.

Wound Healing Team. The team is defining and establishing protocols for appropriate evaluation, intervention, and follow-up of chronic wounds.

Telemetry Team. The team is focusing on ensuring that the utilization of telemetry unit monitoring is appropriate.

Surgical Pathology Reporting Team. The team is working on improving the timeliness of surgical pathology reports.

Source: *Reprinted with permission from Bethesda Hospital, Inc, Cincinnati, Ohio, 1991.*

Case Study
Bethesda's Patient Availability Team

Issue

Delays in patient transportation were a chronic problem at Bethesda North Hospital, and numerous attempts had been made to try to improve the situation. The patient availability team was formed to attempt to reduce delays in the patient transportation system. The team represented a wide range of disciplines, both managers and staff from a number of different departments. Members included

- Dennis Fleming, director of food services and team leader;
- Anne Marie Kaes, critical care nurse;
- Mary Maus, charge nurse;
- Sue Hadley, unit coordinator;
- Lori Tieman, radiology (central scheduling);
- Dave Truesdell, transport;
- Deanna Hoffman, radiology, CT scanner;
- Linda Simbritz, physical therapy;
- John Kennedy, respiratory therapy;
- Timothy Flenner, MD, physical medicine/rehabilitation and physician consultant;
- Ginnie Blocker and Sandy Mazzei, facilitators; and
- John Riefenberger, management engineer.

The manager of management engineering provided invaluable assistance in data gathering and interpretation.

One of the first things we did was identify the team's charge and develop a definition for the problem that it was to address. The team charge became: "Improve communication among ancillary departments and nursing to reduce delays and cancellations at Bethesda North Hospital."

During our initial meetings, all team members believed the solution to the problem was simple—add more patient transporters. The team set out to demonstrate that delays in the system would decrease if more transportation hours were added. We gathered information on the total transports, time of day of transports, day of week of transports, average transportation time, and peak and slow periods of patient transportation. When we examined the total number of productive hours available in the patient transportation system, we discovered that more than enough hours existed. Thus, early in the process, we came to realize that we had to look outside our preconceptions if we wanted to improve the transportation system.

The team charted the patient transportation process from the time that a physician orders a test to the time the patient is returned to his or her room after the ancillary test or service. By plotting the process on a flowchart, we were able to graphically see opportunities for improvement. For example, after the physician's order, we found that it took a total of nine telephone calls to get a patient to his or her test or therapy and back to his or her room. The team soon realized it was almost a miracle we were able to deliver patients to their tests or services, let alone get them there on time.

After developing a cause-and-effect diagram, the team saw that we needed to examine data and determine the causes of delays. We examined delays for inpatient physical therapy exams and delays for inpatient radiology and CT exams. When we looked at the reasons for delays, we found that the most common cause was that the patient was to be discharged. This occurred because nurses did not want to discharge patients until they had completed charting and were unable to chart on discharged patients. The second and third most common reasons for delays were that the patient was eating or in the bathroom. Table 5.A (below) illustrates the causes for delays. The team realized that all these delays were the result of nursing being unable to determine exactly what patients were doing on any given day. (See Figures 5.A–5.C, pages 150–151.)

As a result of the study, the team concurred that the most effective way to increase the efficiency of patient transport was to increase communication among departments. By working with the information systems department, the team found that the patient care plan could be changed so that all the ancillary tests and therapies were printed in red and highlighted. This enabled each patient's nurse to see what that patient was scheduled to do each day. In addition, we discovered that the physical therapy department manually produced a schedule each day. The schedule was typed, duplicated, and distributed to each nursing unit. However, this activity was not complete until after 9:00 AM—a full two hours after the department had begun treating patients.

Table 5.A. Causes for Delay

1. Patient discharged	6. Patient too sick
2. Patient eating	7. Equipment not available
3. Patient in bathroom	8. Patient with physician
4. Patient in another test	9. Patient refused
5. Patient with visitors	10. Other

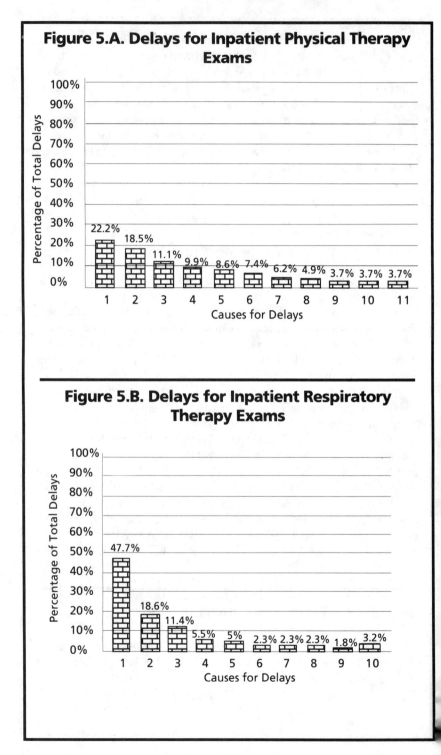

Figure 5.A. Delays for Inpatient Physical Therapy Exams

Figure 5.B. Delays for Inpatient Respiratory Therapy Exams

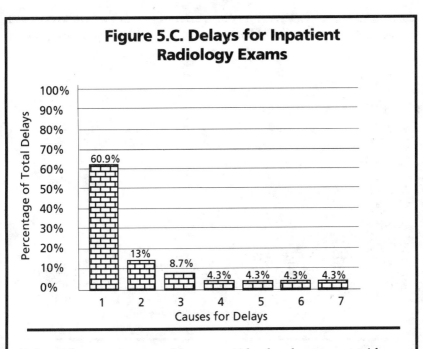

Figure 5.C. Delays for Inpatient Radiology Exams

Information systems was able to provide the department with an electronic blackboard enabling them to type the physical therapy schedule each day and have it automatically transmitted to each nursing unit.

The team discovered that the number one problem was a result of the nursing staff's inability to chart on a patient who had left their unit (see Figure 5.D, page 152). Information systems was able to change the access capabilities for each nurse enabling them to chart on their patients up to 24 hours after they had been transferred from the unit.

As a result of our analysis of peaks and flows in the patient transportation system, we made schedule adjustments for the patient transporters. Prior to studying the patient availability issue, there were only three starting times for transporters. The supervisor of patient transport has now staggered his schedule to ensure that there are sufficient transporters available to handle the peaks in the demand.

As a result of data-gathering activities and brainstorming sessions, the team developed standard protocols for the way unit coordinators would be educated to properly order tests.

We also demonstrated that the radiology department and central scheduling would better meet the needs of patients if we expanded their hours. In order to decrease the number of telephone calls in the transportation process, the team recommended that the hospital purchase two-way radios, which would be carried by each transporter and

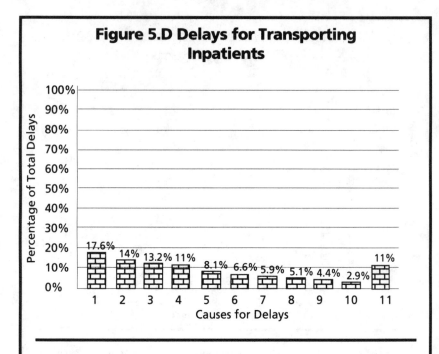

Figure 5.D Delays for Transporting Inpatients

linked to a central patient dispatcher. This new system resulted in a decrease in the number of telephone calls to a total of four and immediate access for the dispatcher to every patient transporter.

Following the implementation of our recommendations, the team noted a dramatic increase in the effectiveness and the satisfaction with patient transport. Six months after all the measures were put into place, the team conducted a two-week follow-up study to determine the degree of customer satisfaction. We were pleased to discover that several original causes of delay had been entirely eliminated: the patient to be discharged and the patient eating or in the bathroom. We also conducted an in-depth evaluation of customer satisfaction with the process. The ancillary departments, radiology, physical therapy, and respiratory therapy, indicated that delays in transport were no longer a major factor in the operation of those departments. We continue to monitor daily delays in the transportation system. (See Figure 5.E, page 153). This is a function of the patient transport dispatcher and supervisor. The data is gathered to ensure that the process is kept within acceptable, predetermined limits. This information is also used to adjust the transporter's schedules when necessary.

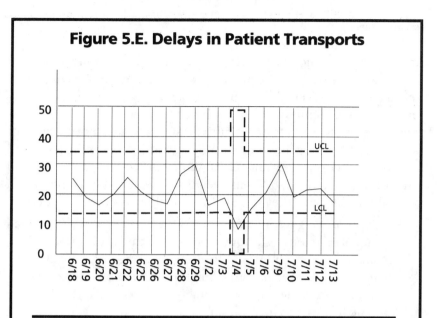

Figure 5.E. Delays in Patient Transports

Evaluation

We have reduced the stretcher transport time within the hospital by approximately 33% and reduced the wheelchair transport time by 42%. The cost of the radio transport system was approximately $10,000. The system more than paid for itself in its first six months of operation in that we chose not to add additional patient transport hours, which would have cost approximately $18,000-$24,000 per year. A list of exams that a patient is scheduled for now prints on the nursing care plan and is an effective tool in helping nurses plan their patients' care.

The team's success was a result of the hard work of all the team members. Each member came to believe that he or she was a force in shaping process improvements at Bethesda Hospital. The team believed that their efforts significantly improved the process and will result in higher quality care to patients and better service to all customers.

Source: *Written by Dennis Fleming, Manager, Physician Relations and Outreach Services (previously Director of Bethesda North's Food Service) and the Patient Availability Team Leader, Bethesda Hospital, Inc, Cincinnati, Ohio, 1991.*

(continued from page 146)

With each new round of teams, Kaminski and the Steering Committee refine the project team process based on the lessons they learn from past rounds. For example, after one round, staff realized that teams needed a direct link to management. A sponsor—the member of senior management closest to the process being investigated—is now assigned to each team. While the sponsor does not necessarily attend each meeting, he or she serves as an advocate for the team and a liaison with the Steering Committee, providing resources and guidance when needed. Team leaders and facilitators identified several other lessons they have learned in their team experiences:

- At first, teams gave interim reports on their activities to a small group of selected staff. Now the doors are thrown open for senior management and other staff to attend and to give feedback to the team. This new approach has heightened visibility and communication. "It's much more informal," one team member said. "More people feel free to give comments."

- The Steering Committee now allows teams to determine their own meeting schedule and time frames for completion. Initial teams were required to meet for eight hours a week, to allow sufficient time for team meetings and education, and were given specific time frames for completing their investigations.

- Enthusiasm at Bethesda is limited by the number of facilitators. "There are a thousand great ideas for teams and only so many facilitators," Kaminski says. She hopes that now that they have begun training managers as additional facilitators, they will eventually be able to support more team activity, both formal and informal.

Bethesda's teams are also asked to identify barriers that are common across the organization, such as charges that were too large and a preference for learning in a just-in-time fashion.

Mini teams. As division and department managers become familiar with Hoshin planning, they are pulling together teams to investigate problems they uncover through the planning process. The processes these mini teams look at are smaller in scope than those being addressed by the cross-functional teams, Kaminski said. They work at a comparatively fast pace, completing their investigation in eight to ten sessions. For example, a mini team in the Bethesda North ambulatory surgery center was formed to study and make improvements that would decrease the number of times a patient's surgery is cancelled without the ambulatory surgery center knowing of the cancellation prior to the scheduled time of surgery. As described in "Education," mini teams receive an abbreviated training format. Kaminski views the mini teams as a "quick way of introducing staff and getting them interested in tools and methods," but she understands there is a trade-off. "The facilitator does most of the work because the pace is so fast," she says. These mini teams help maintain the enthusiasm generated for TQM as staff are taught the concepts and tools.

Department teams. As a part of daily management, many departments across the organization are forming teams to deal with an issue specific to their department. For example, the Bethesda Oak radiology department is improving the process of retrieving previously read x-ray films requested by attending physicians.

In a departure from traditional problem solving, Bethesda is now piloting a new type of team in the alcohol/drug department that operates solely according to Nadler's seven principles of breakthrough thinking.[2] While they are just beginning to experiment with this approach, Kaminski distinguishes projects they would approach using breakthrough thinking from those they would approach with their 13-step model. Nadler's ideas are used when totally revising a system or creating a new system, rather than putting an existing process "under a microscope," Kaminski says. For example, the alcohol and drug treatment project's goal is "to design a plan to maximize individualized treatment provided to patients, given the available resources." The emphasis is on design rather than dissection to achieve process improvement. Breakthrough thinking is a more creative method than traditional problem-solving, which is more quantitative and analytical. Breakthrough thinking is also less methodical; team members do not follow a sequential application of the seven breakthrough thinking principles in a step-by-step approach. Kaminski describes breakthrough thinking as more of a "branching," nonlinear process in which the team often arrives at "four different paradigms or alternative systems."

QA/QI Relationship

QA staff feel the current emphasis on TQM is helpful to them since management and staff will pay even more attention to data and information, according to Larry Johnstal, QA director. Staff have already begun to use TQM tools (for example, control charts, Pareto diagrams) to present traditional QA data, and QA findings often instigate the formation of quality improvement teams to investigate a process. The hospital is currently developing a plan that will incorporate the positive attributes of both QA and QI.

Education

Kaminski stresses that a TQM organization has to have a climate "that supports learning" since "you will be continually telling your staff to learn from mistakes." Bethesda appropriated funds to support the organization's emphasis on learning. The total direct dollar investment between 1988 and the end of 1991 (four budget years) is projected at approximately $860,000. A major part of this expense (over $400,000) was money allocated to replace staff when they were participating on a team or attending training during the first two years of the roll out.

With a strong history of education before TQM (for example, courses were provided in customer service education and management/leadership skills), Bethesda was fortunate to have a core group of professional educators to help deploy TQM throughout the organization and to rewrite GOAL/QPC materials so they were specific to health care and Bethesda. The hospital has also been able to capitalize on the management engineering department, which provided statistical expertise even before Bethesda committed to TQM. The engineers were "the external experts coming into the department doing consulting," Kaminski says. "Now departments use the tools on their own," and the engineers serve primarily as consultants to teams and facilitators (for example, helping them devise accurate control charts). "The organization may have to put up with less precise statistical analysis for awhile," Kaminski says, "but the trade-off is investment of people in the process."

Management struggled at first with the role management engineering should play in the roll out of TQM. Wilburn decided to deploy TQM through corporate education based on early conversations with Kaminski in which they concurred it would be more effective for nonstatisticians to teach the tools. Most of the instructors in corporate education are former nurses, dieticians, and other health care professionals. "The only way to get people to learn these tools is if Nancy Glorious in her nursing hat teaches them," Kaminski says. "If employees see that regular staff can learn and use these tools and teach the tools themselves, it sends a powerful message that you don't have to be an industrial engineer to learn the tools."

Bethesda's education approach is based on theories of adult education that say "people learn more effectively when they have a need for the information and can use it immediately," Kaminski says. While everyone in the organization has received awareness training (that is, Quality 1 overview) that introduces them to the concepts of Deming and Bethesda's 13-step process improvement model, instruction in the tools, Hoshin, daily management, and so forth are taught on a just-in-time basis. Formal TQM-related education has been developed and is managed under the leadership of Maureen Hollenbeck, head of human resource development and TQM education department, and includes the following:

- Quality 1 awareness course, which is provided to everyone in the organization.

- Team training, which is provided based on the type of team:

  —Each round of Quality 1 teams receives a two-day training course that includes an overview of TQM at Bethesda, instruction on the 13-step model and CQI tools, and a team-building session. During the second day the teams actually hold their first meeting and during the remainder of the process they receive just-in-time education on the seven quality control tools.

  —Mini teams receive an abridged version of the two-day education cross-functional teams receive, which lasts about 30-45 minutes. The facilitator often takes on the role of leader on these teams, and provides just-in-time training as necessary.

  —Department teams receive either the abridged or regular education depending on their needs and the scope of their project.

- Team leaders receive 1 ½ days of education before they join their teams. After the training, they are able to describe TQM philosophy, walk their teams through the use of at least five tools, and organize and conduct a team meeting.

- Sponsors undergo a 16-hour course after which they understand the sponsor role, are able to discuss no-fault learning and how to model it, understand their role in giving and receiving feedback, and so on.

- Facilitator education occurs in two phases, a basic course (five days) and an advanced course (three days).

- All new managers receive a 1 ½-day management orientation, which includes an introduction to Deming and the Bethesda management approach.

- A 48-hour course begun before Bethesda became committed to TQM, "Leadership: Imagine the Possibilities" is a program based on the Zenger-Miller "Supervision" program, which includes such topics as listening, resolving conflict, counseling on employee problems, hiring effectively, solving problems creatively, and overcoming resistance to change. Since TQM was adopted at the hospital, the course has been revised so it weaves TQM concepts throughout. Every manager at Bethesda, from charge nurse to executive, completes this course.

An important element of Bethesda's education is that Wilburn discusses Quality 1 concepts at all corporate orientation sessions. A specific orientation session is mandatory for all employees. In addition, all newly hired or promoted managers are required to participate in a 1 ½-day management orientation. Wilburn also speaks to every round of teams during their education. At the Quality 1 overview, either Wilburn or a senior vice-president spends an hour responding to questions of staff. Management members of the Quality 1 Steering Committee are currently involved with teams as sponsors, leaders, and members.

QI Supports

Crucial to rolling out Bethesda's TQM approach has been the establishment of an effective support network that includes a sophisticated information system and comprehensive customer tracking system.

Customer-supplier feedback structure. Besides facilitating QFD teams (see page 136), marketing is intensely gathering qualitative and quantitative feedback from customers. The methods they use (for example, surveys, focus groups) are specific to each of the five customer groups the Steering Committee identified. For example, the department tracks patient and physician satisfaction using the following methods:

- *Patients.* Before TQM, patients were mailed a survey after they left the hospital. Although the hospital had a 15% response rate, marketing suspected the data they received were biased (that is, only patients who were either pleased or unhappy with service were returning the surveys). They decided to adopt a telephone survey instead and contracted with the Gallup Organization, in Princeton, New Jersey, to randomly interview 8%–10% of the patients discharged from Bethesda. Patients are asked rating questions (for example, on a scale of 1 to 4 how would you rate the hospital environment?) and open-ended questions (for example, what kind of things would make your stay better?). Marketing is continually "exploring how to word the questions in order to get appropriate feedback that will help us better understand patient expectations," Stacey says. It has also been "hard to get patients to identify what's important to them," says Tom Ferguson, senior vice-president, corporate services. Instead they "found it easier to ask what is expected . . . [patients] want safe care, but they won't say it because that's expected."

The Gallup Organization provides formal reports including narrative, graphs, and tables twice a year. Individual reports are also prepared for specific departments. The hospital is developing "service quality" indices that will allow the organization to track and monitor their performance over time. These indices can be categorized into one of five areas: assurance, empathy, reliability, responsiveness, and tangibles.

- *Physicians.* To achieve the hospital's objective of becoming the preferred place for physicians to practice, marketing has been working closely with Professional Research Consultants, an independent research firm, to survey both medical staff members and referring physicians to determine what they consider a "quality" hospital. They proceeded with the medical staff in two phases. A focus group was held to gather qualitative data, which were then used to design a telephone survey to attain follow-up quantitative information. The quantitative results showed that medical staff members gave the highest importance to a responsive nursing staff, the delivery of prompt patient care, good radiology services, a well-trained medical staff, and good lab services. They gave the least importance to the convenience of location to their office and educational opportunities. Marketing is presently gathering findings from telephone interviews with referring physicians.

In addition to the general medical staff study, clinical teams are researching customer needs to drive the process improvements. For example, physicians who use the telemetry unit were interviewed by physician representatives to understand their needs for usage and desired enhancements of services," said Weinstein. The fertility center team used marketing to conduct focus groups with patients. The results caused the team to become sensitized to the emotional and service needs of the patients. Marketing also helps Quality 1 teams and other departments collect customer feedback to validate customer needs.

Information system. Significant to Bethesda's TQM efforts is the addition of an integrated Executive Information System (EIS), being developed in conjunction with MEDICUS, that will assist top management with the TQM process and will include data on the ten critical measures as well as Hoshin planning, daily management, team activities, and QFD projects. For example, the EIS will allow managers to access control charts on their terminals that reflect whether the "results reporting time by department process" (one of Bethesda's ten critical measures) is in control. For daily management, EIS aggregates outcome data from various sources in order to measure an entire process (for example, patient encounters can be linked to episodes of the processes a patient goes through). For Hoshin planning, EIS defines the organization hierarchically and can look at data on the achievement of goals at any level of the top of the organization. EIS will eventually be able to track Joint Commission indicators and compliance with standards.

The majority of the Bethesda data systems—patient care, financial, medical record, billing, and EIS—are automated and interface with each other. This will enable the information systems division to provide the process-oriented data needed by Quality 1 teams and to provide senior management with access to information for planning and tracking. With approximately 350 personal computers and 650 computer terminals, staff throughout the organization can access needed information.

Since Bethesda began its TQM effort, the work load of the information systems division has increased 20%; staff from the department participate on teams either as full members or consultants, and information services receives recommendations from teams on needed system changes. Statistical software allows teams to create control charts, flowcharts, cause-and-effect diagrams, and other TQM tools on their computers; however, as part of adult education concerns, team members are usually required to create these manually.

Reward and recognition. Interested in revising their present merit system to reflect TQM principles, staff in human resources are presently assessing the consistency of Bethesda's policies with Deming's 14 points using a matrix. The school of nursing is also working on alternatives to performance evaluations that might be applicable across the hospital. In 1989, the board also installed a long-term incentive plan for senior management based on quality management and linked to quality objectives. This plan replaced a short-term focused cash incentive program based on market share improvements. Staff are recognized for their work on teams with a participation pin, and they have regular discussions with management. Bethesda does not have an employee of the month award or a quality day because management feels these would give the message the TQM was separate from daily activities and would stress competition instead of teamwork and cooperation.

An important instrument that human resources uses in monitoring employee satisfaction is the employee opinion survey designed by Management Science Associates. The survey provides feedback that can be aggregated in 16 key topic areas. Employees evaluate such statements as "efficiency is highly valued in my department," "I often go home after work with a feeling of satisfaction about my job," and "quality is a top priority at Bethesda." The current employee opinion survey has been conducted biannually and is being redesigned to monitor employee satisfaction more frequently. A new section has recently been added to the survey that will help management determine what aspects of staff's jobs are the most important in making Bethesda the preferred place to work in Cincinnati—one of their breakthrough objectives.

Supplier relationships. As a shareholder in the American Healthcare System (AMHS), an alliance of 40 systems composed of 1,200 hospitals, Bethesda benefits from the long-term group buying agreements AMHS has established with major corporations, many of whom are involved in TQM, such as 3M, Johnson & Johnson, Fuji, and IBM. While the buying agreements are negotiated at the AMHS level, each hospital develops its own relationships with the companies. This establishes a partnership through which they work toward mutual benefits. The long-term agreements have allowed Bethesda to establish relationships with these suppliers and involve them in quality improvement initiatives. A Johnson & Johnson employee is a member of Bethesda's wound closure product team. Other efforts with suppliers include working with DuPont to smooth out the ordering process so that Bethesda's inventory remains low and DuPont's production can be more regular and setting up a benchmarking system through Baxter and the AMHS for hospitals to study the best practices in material management. Staff are expecting to begin selecting vendors based on their quality activities and look at ways to decrease variation in the products they receive.

Benchmarking. During its initial development, the Steering Committee compared approaches through the National Demonstration Project and studied more mature industries such as Procter & Gamble, IBM, Xerox, and others. A Japanese professor well versed in TQM paid a visit to Bethesda early on. Teams are also benchmarking. For example, the asthma care team called a national referral center and local emergency departments to determine their standards of care before developing Bethesda's standards and offering in-service training for all Bethesda facilities on the proper care process.

Physician Involvement

One consultant who visited Bethesda early in their TQM effort advised Wilburn to begin by looking at the admitting and billing processes. Wilburn reacted against this advice remembering his early attempts to use manufacturing methods in health care. "No one is going to remember you for having the best registration system," Wilburn says. "You should have it, but it is not the [most important part of the] business we're in." Instead Bethesda began involving the medical staff in TQM from the beginning. After a medical staff retreat in April 1989, several physician leaders volunteered to serve on the Quality 1 medical staff advisory group. Since then the advisory group has received extensive training in TQM concepts and tools, and selected projects to pilot test TQM in medicine. One project they piloted, the asthma treatment team, helped prove that TQM could effect change in physician practice patterns and develop consistent systems for diagnosing and treating patients.

Presently Weinstein is beginning to introduce TQM to a larger segment of the medical staff in several ways: introducing TQM concepts at medical staff department meetings; encouraging physicians to use TQM in the management of their offices (for example, a neurosurgeon and a radiation oncologist have been using TQM in their group practices); developing physician-specific education materials; devoting parts of, or entire, physician retreats to TQM; inviting an expert who specializes in clinical TQM to present the results; and involving more medical staff on teams. Weinstein is approaching the time dilemma physicians face with TQM by involving physicians as consultants on cross-functional teams that look at administrative

162

processes and as full members and/or leaders on clinical mini teams.

While Weinstein and Kaminski have found that "the same issues come up in educating physicians as when educating other staff" on TQM, Weinstein identifies some of these issues when tying medical staff involvement to Bethesda's core concepts:

- *Continuous improvement.* "Medicine has a foundation in quality improvement," Weinstein says. She points to the difference with TQM. "You're not looking for the bad apple physician but shifting to improved performance of the whole group."

- *Customer.* "Customer" is a barrier word for physicians (that is, patients as customers), according to Weinstein. "Physicians have difficulty communicating in the language of TQM," agrees Paul Lewis, MD, president, medical staff.

- *Variation.* Physicians immediately see the application in nonclinical areas (for example, inconsistency in stat lab). "They refer to it as 'hassle reducer,'" Weinstein says. However, controversy erupts when discussion turns to understanding variation in clinical practice, she says. Bethesda is attempting to shift physician attitudes. For example, Brent James, MD, recently spoke to the medical staff on improving clinical results through TQM. The hospital is piloting studies in total hip and knee replacement and cesarian sections.

- *Teamwork.* "Understanding the complexity involved in the system of care [which is discovered through teamwork] is an important . . . learning process for physicians through participation on teams," Weinstein said.

Conclusion

Transforming a culture takes a mix of courage and caution. While Wilburn and his staff are anxious to see the results of their TQM initiatives, they understand the value of patience. "We're a risk-taking organization," Wilburn said, "but generally we have some data in hand before undertaking it." This philosophy is reflected in the hospital's approach to TQM. With an innovative information system, a sophisticated customer tracking system, and Japanese-proven planning strategies such as Hoshin planning, Bethesda will be able to monitor each new addition to its "house of quality."

References

1. GOAL/QPC: *Total Quality Management Implementation Health Care Services Manual.* Methuen, MA, 1989.

2. Nadler G, Hibino S: *Breakthrough Thinking.* Rocklin, CA: Prima Publishing & Communications. 1990, pp 6-10.

3. King B: *Hoshin Planning. The Developmental Approach.* Methuen, MA: GOAL/QPC, 1989.

4. Brassard M: *The Memory Jogger Plus, Featuring the Seven Management and Planning Tools.* Methuen, MA: GOAL/QPC, 1989.

5. Moran J, Collett C, Core C: *Daily Management.* Methuen, MA: GOAL/QPC, 1989.

6. GOAL/QPC: *Memory Jogger. A Pocket Guide of Tools for Continuous Improvement.* Methuen, MA: GOAL/QPC, 1988.

7. King B: *Better Designs in Half the Time: Implementing Quality Function Deployment (QFD).* Methuen, MA: GOAL/QPC, 1989.

6 Looking Beyond Classic TQM

Strong Memorial Hospital at the University of Rochester
Rochester, New York

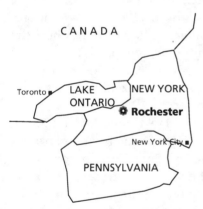

CANADA

Toronto

LAKE ONTARIO

Rochester

NEW YORK

New York City

PENNSYLVANIA

Type of hospital: Academic medical center
Scope of services: General medical/surgical
Beds: 715, with an average census of 622
Extent of TQM involvement: Strong began investigating quality improvement methods as part of the National Demonstration Project in 1988. All senior management are trained, several teams are making progress, and management is beginning to cascade TQM through the organization using Xerox's "family" approach to training. Simultaneously, Strong is pursuing the improvement of clinical processes through a hospitalwide research program, "Innovations in Patient Care"

Special aspects of Strong's TQM activities:
— Innovations in Patient Care program that is addressing clinical process improvement
— Emphasis on research as method to move toward TQM
— Communitywide interest in and pressure toward using quality improvement measures
— Tight industry connection, particularly with Baldrige winner Xerox
— Member of academic medical consortium moving toward outcomes management as a tool for TQM
— Development of early TQM support in medical and nursing schools

When speaking about total quality management (TQM), senior executives at Strong always preface it with an adjective (for example, "classic" TQM), suggesting there is another type of TQM. Making a distinction between clinical process improvement and clinical *support* process improvement, Paul Griner, MD, general director, and Leo Brideau, executive director, consider Strong to be in the early stages of "classic" TQM, or the improvement of support processes (for example, admissions, pharmacy) but feel the hospital is advancing rapidly along a second track—clinical process improvement—which has sprung out of Strong's Innovations in Patient Care (IPC) program.[1,2] For the fifth year, Strong is funding independent research projects that hospital physicians, nurses, and clinicians propose to improve patient care and/or reduce costs. The IPC program has funded 45 studies in all and paid for itself several times over in the first year alone. Bob Panzer, MD, director, office of clinical practice evaluation, sees the IPC as a tool for use in TQM to improve clinical outputs. Another distinction that leaders at Strong make is that "classic TQM," as implemented in many health care institutions, needs to be extended further in academic medical centers, where the scope of TQM needs to address community, regional, and national issues and the tools need to encompass research and education. "Deming gave us the 14 points 30 years ago," Panzer says, "now there is a need to take the TQM model further."

Strong was already into "the fabric of TQM" and didn't know it, according to Wilbur Pittman of Xerox, who is chairman of Strong's board. The hospital's culture is one that many would consider a product of TQM: high respect for the individual, systems thinking, appreciation for new ideas, and empowerment at the line level. Brideau says "there is a kind of gentility" at Strong. When he arrived at the hospital eleven years ago, he got the sense that he was "charged with preserving a treasure." Understanding the culture at Strong involves looking at the unique history of both the medical center and the community of Rochester. One clue is the approach to patient care emphasized at the medical school. George Hoyt Whipple, first dean of the medical school, emphasized approaching patient care holistically—a unique concept back in 1926 when the school opened. Today the medical school continues to focus on elements of medicine within a broader context, extending beyond the classroom and research laboratory. Students work with health care mentors and as volunteers in schools and community agencies, which allows them to see the provision of medicine within a systems context. In addition to respect for the patient, the hospital promotes respect for all members of the health care team and the contributions they make. The medical school considers the unique value of each applicant's potential contribution to the school and does not require MCAT scores. "There is a fertile environment at Strong," says John Olivier, senior director for patient care programs. "People who work here are accustomed to . . . investigating new ideas. Quality is not just a concept at Strong, it has long been part of the culture."

Another clue to Strong's cooperative culture is the Rochester Area Hospital Corporation, an umbrella organization through which the six area hospitals in Rochester work together to reduce costs and increase quality and access throughout the region. Since its inception ten years ago, "health care costs in Rochester, New York, have come in a full 25% below the rise in the national average."[3] During a time when most hospitals across the country were becoming more competitive, Strong and other Rochester hospitals were working together. For example, a single $2 1/4 million kidney lithotripter, a state-of-the-art technology in kidney stone treatment, was purchased for use by physicians throughout the region. Rather than each hospital purchasing its own, Strong acquired the region's lithotripter and granted all qualified urologists in the area restricted privileges to the lithotripter facility. A second arrangement grants area cardiologists limited privileges to the area's two cardiac catheterization units, which are located at Strong and Rochester General Hospital. Under this arrangement, cardiologists don't have to worry about losing patients to cardiologists with regular privileges at Strong or Rochester General.[4] "Friends tell me I'm in never-never land . . . that community planning doesn't happen like this elsewhere," says Susan Powell, director of clinical support services. Rather than stress market competition, "Paul [Griner] and Leo [Brideau] have stressed the larger agenda and support a network of high-quality hospitals in Rochester," Powell says.

Rochester Area Hospital Corporation is a by-product of the heightened sense of community responsibility present in Rochester. Business leaders became involved in health care planning as far back as the 1930s when they agreed to make Blue Cross/Blue Shield the principal health insurer and to community-rate all employee insurance. Over fifty years later, "the average annual Blue Cross/Blue Shield premium in Rochester for 1990 was just over $1,600. The national . . . average was $3,500."[5] In the 1960s when hospitals across the country were adding more beds, business and community leaders in Rochester came together to research the number of beds needed throughout the region before allocating funds toward that end.

Currently, Strong and other Rochester area hospitals are uniting again with local industries in a "Partnership for Quality." After reviewing a number of options, the hospitals have agreed that the most promising way to assure their goal of quality services at low costs and high access is to fully implement TQM across all six hospitals in a partnership with local industry. All six hospitals are beginning or advancing TQM efforts within their individual institutions, and they have all committed to collaborative TQM efforts at the community level. For example, hospitals may address the chronic problem of a heavy influx of patients to emergency rooms that exceeds their capacity. The community efforts will be guided by a Partnership for Quality Committee, which will be made up of industry and hospital leaders. Fortunate to have Eastman Kodak and Xerox (a recent winner of the Malcolm Baldrige award) within the city limits, the hospitals will be able to draw on the experiences these companies have had in implementing TQM.

Description and Demographics

Innovation is inherent to the culture of Rochester. Related to population, more than three times as many patents are granted to Rochester area residents than the rest of the country.[6] Such industry giants as Xerox and Eastman Kodak were founded here, and Rochester is generally considered the imaging and optics capital of the world. Located in upstate New York near Lake Ontario, Rochester's population is approximately one million in the metropolitan area. Rochester's economy has remained stable over the years; at the end of the recent recession, unemployment peaked at 5.4%. Even in the 1980s when Xerox had to lay off 12,000 people, most workers who chose not to retire were quickly swept up by the small technological firms multiplying around the city.

With over 700 beds, Strong is the largest of the six hospitals in Rochester. An academic medical center and referral center for a nine-county area, Strong has all major specialties, with special expertise in orthopaedic medicine, cardiac care, transplantation medicine, and cancer care, and serves as the regional center for burn care, trauma, and perinatal care. The medical center, which includes the hospital, the School of Medicine and Dentistry, and the School of Nursing, is part of the University of Rochester, a private university with 8,233 students. While the rest of the medical center has not made a formal move to TQM, Strong deals with university departments and components in their role as "vendors of services," Brideau says. He believes that over time other elements of the university will embrace TQM.

History

Before making the commitment to TQM, a culture that supported TQM concepts was developing at Strong. For example, the IPC program encouraged innovation and research. As explained further in "Philosophy," the success of the IPC program has affected the mindsets of many clinicians throughout the medical center and university. While IPC projects have not specifically used TQM tools and methods, the scientific principles and methods that parallel TQM methods are employed. Applicants are encouraged to undertake studies in five priority areas, and systems improvement is now one of these areas. Another component of the hospital's antecedent culture was the move to matrix management in 1982. Major programs are managed by a team that includes a physician, nursing chiefs of service, other clinical leaders, and a professional administrator; this emphasizes collaboration among the disciplines. "TQM supports [the antecedents]," Brideau says. "The underlying culture is a passion for making it better, to let a number of mechanisms flourish if they are improving the quality of the organization."

Strong began formally exploring TQM methods as one of the original participants in the National Demonstration Project. In 1987 staff formed a team to reduce waiting times in the emergency department. After several months of data collection and investigation, which included hiring students to determine with stopwatches where patients spent the majority of their "wait" time, the team was able to narrow the problem down to several specific causes. Causes of delays fell into two major categories: delays in patient registration, which were addressed through cross-training and changes in responsibility, and delays in clinical evaluation, which were addressed through increased attending physician intervention (for example, setting priorities and expediting the care process). Although some of the interventions to reduce waiting time were not implemented until two years later (due to leadership turnover), Brideau feels the experience was worthwhile since the team "taught us a lot about quality improvement tools and methods."

The beginning of Strong's TQM effort suffered from many stops and starts. Just as senior management were getting their feet wet, the hospitals in New York State were hit with a major budget crisis. As in the rest of the country, labor costs rose rapidly in 1988 and 1989 due to significant labor shortages. New York State, which sets rates for all nonfederal payers, failed to fully recognize these increased costs in hospital reimbursement rates. This shortfall coupled with a small projected downturn in patient volumes forced Strong to make a $14 million adjustment to its 1989 budget. Senior management were hesitant to begin a large scale commitment to TQM at this time because TQM "would have been associated with cost cutting rather than quality," Brideau says. The hospital had to delay their TQM efforts for a year until the budget was under control. Looking back, Brideau feels it was probably "wise to stop and assess" their direction back in 1989 because of "the little education" management had at the time. However, he says "it would be disastrous" to stop their TQM effort now two years after making a commitment.

In 1990 the hospital explored a joint venture with a component of the Rochester Institute of Technology (RIT), a local university that has a background in teaching and consulting on TQM to manufacturing industries. Staff hoped RIT could contribute TQM and statistical knowledge and Strong would provide the health care experience. Pilot teams began using representatives from RIT as consultants. While helpful because of the lessons learned, these initial teams suffered setbacks. Other than the small number of staff involved on teams, very few people at Strong were aware of TQM and teams were forced to work in relative isolation. They had difficulty recruiting staff to collect data and implement their proposals. Strong's teams also had to spend the first several months helping the consultant understand health care issues instead of using him as a trainer. Brideau cautions that "a consultant is not going to put TQM into place for your organization. You must go through a gestational period, you have to grow on your own."

A galvanizing step for Strong was a site visit to Xerox. Senior managers visited top management at Xerox and learned how TQM is used in daily activities. The site visit made staff "rethink [their] ways," Brideau says. Senior management are now focusing on planning and building a core understanding of TQM throughout the hospital rather than rapidly multiplying the number of teams. At approximately the same time that Strong began reexamining its approach, many members of the National Demonstration Project and its Quality

Management Network began to rethink their strategy. "It seemed that some of us [in the Quality Management Network] were getting caught up in the 'How many project teams do you have?' contest," Jeanne Dent remembers. "What happened was that teams knew the tools and techniques but couldn't talk to others in the organization." Strong's change in direction coincided with a greater emphasis on planning on the part of many members of the Quality Management Network.

A Steering Committee made up of senior management was organized to oversee Strong's TQM effort. Brideau has overall responsibility for TQM at the hospital, and a Quality Resources Group has been organized, which includes facilitators, trainers, and internal consultants to support the rollout. Approximately 20 staff members have been trained as facilitators.

Strong's board is very supportive of the hospital's TQM efforts, and many members are involved in TQM through their own businesses. Board members have become involved in hospital quality activities first-hand through the board quality of care committee. "It is important that the board is dead serious about quality...." Brideau says, telling the story of how Pittman schedules all his other activities around hospital activities. The first dates Pittman marks on his calendar each January are the hospital board and quality-of-care meetings.

Coinciding with Strong's overall TQM initiative, the office of clinical practice evaluation (OCPE) began its own intensive TQM activities. As the internal research department that oversees the IPC program and other clinical analysis activities, the OCPE has a lot of linkages throughout the hospital, and the department's TQM activities have begun to inspire others. According to Panzer, he and his staff "couldn't wait the two years for it [TQM] to cascade down" the organization. Since it is an isolated department, which is actually located in a building separate from the hospital, Panzer and his staff got permission to begin TQM in their department at their own pace. Since then, the department has set up its own Quality Improvement Council, begun several project teams, and developed its own vision to "be a national leader in clinical practice analysis and research in support of Strong." While Brideau supports the excitement created by OCPE's TQM activities, he warns "you can't create a culture ... with uncontrolled diversity." One lesson Brideau learned from Xerox is to use the same training manual, the same language, and so on when attempting a cultural transformation. Since the OCPE is geographically isolated from the rest of the hospital, Brideau does not worry about the department's activities contradicting the culture that the hospital is creating and supports its efforts.

Since their visit to Xerox, members of senior management have undergone extensive training in TQM concepts and methods. An important part of their education has been using the techniques themselves to devise strategy. Top management formed into two teams. One team devised the hospital's TQM implementation plan, and the other is redesigning a process for the approval and support of new projects. Other hospitals have begun to be trained in peer groups using Xerox's "family" method (for example, program management teams attend training together). Brideau worries that the hospital will suffer a lag period until training is completed since staff will have varying levels of TQM knowledge. "We don't want to make a big splash announcement [about TQM] when the line employee may not get trained for two years," Brideau says. However, as discussed in "Strategy," senior managers are being encouraged to use TQM methods without fanfare in daily activities so "staff will get used to the language and concepts," Brideau says.

Philosophy

Taking advantage of the research and educational capabilities they have on site, senior management members plan to deploy these resources in defining the scope of "maximal" quality improvement. As an academic medical center, senior management at Strong envision their TQM activities stretching beyond "classical" TQM. Brideau and Panzer challenge that "total" quality management should be, in fact, total. They insist that if boundaries or limitations are placed on where TQM might be applied, then "maximal" improvement will not be reached. The boundaries of TQM are already being tested at Strong through the IPC program and cooperative efforts in the community. Understanding that academic leaders will be skeptical of efforts focusing only on administrative or support activities, senior management are encouraging the investigations being conducted through the IPC program into clinical systems improvement.

The medical school has always emphasized basic research, but the IPC program funds applied health services research—how to deliver better patient care. The success of the IPC program generating new knowledge, improving care, and saving money shows how applied health services research compliments and often operationalizes basic biomedical research. For example, a first-year study by Ann McMullen, RN, determined that an inexpensive saline solution could maintain patency in the small catheters used for intermittent intravenous access as effectively as the more expensive heparin. This conclusion has saved Strong about $70,000 each year.[2] In another study, researchers from the department of pediatrics, led by Kathleen Wooden, MD, were able to reduce the length of stay (a total of 109 days avoided for 73 patients for a cost savings of $20,165) in children with serious infections. Her study showed no decrease in clinical outcomes for patients discharged early when they were provided with daily intramuscular Ceftriaxone at home. From the perspective of the children and their families, being able to stay at home is seen as an improvement in care delivery. Successes such as these in applied health services research have increased the number of faculty in the medical and nursing schools who want to conduct research in hospital services.

Beyond stretching the boundaries of TQM within the hospital, members of senior management also envision their TQM activities extending beyond the walls of the institution. As an academic medical center, staff feel a responsibility to contribute to improving the health of the community and providing research that has national and international impact. Efforts are beginning through Rochester Area Hospital Corporation to address root causes of communitywide health concerns. For example, Panzer emphasizes that excellent neonatal care is not "maximal" quality when a lack of prenatal care has resulted in some of the premature babies that need to be cared for in neonatal intensive care units.

Strategy

Strong's five-year strategic plan has seven goals that will help the hospital achieve its mission of "improving the health of residents of the Finger Lakes region and upstate New York by providing high-quality patient care services. . . ." TQM is the first goal. Each year, senior management develop a management plan that spells out specific objectives and tasks under each goal. For example, in the 1991 management plan, tasks under TQM include providing orientation to medical clinical chiefs, developing a plan for integrating benchmarking as a routine management tool, and customizing their quality manual and training tools. Crucial in developing their TQM strategy was the assessment of Strong's culture and environment. The Steering Committee completed the exercise in Figure 6.1 (pages 174–175) before determining their strategic objectives.

One important task the hospital hopes to accomplish in 1991 is the

An Exercise for Organizational Assessment

An environment in which there is no organized, widely recognized and respected system for reward and recognition for employees	1 2 3 4 5	An environment in which an organized and respected reward system exists and attracts wide employee participation
An environment in which management members have too many projects with no method of prioritizing them	1 2 3 4 5	An environment in which management members are able to manage their many projects, based on a priority system in which all members participate
An environment in which the tools necessary to measure the improvement quality is difficult and virtually nonexistent	1 2 3 4 5	An environment in which the tools to measure improvement in in quality exist in our environment and are used routinely
An environment in which an excessive focus on academics can produce a preoccupation with analysis and delay decision making	1 2 3 4 5	An environment in which data and analysis are utilized to expedite/ facilitate decision making
An environment where risk taking is discouraged. A culture which subtly promotes avoidance of difficult problems	1 2 3 4 5	An environment in which wise risk taking is encouraged, particularly when such action involves an attempt to address difficult problems
An environment in which there is an incomplete or ambiguous understanding of customer requirements	1 2 3 4 5	An environment in which a systematic approach is used to understand and satisfy both internal and external customer requirements
An environment in which individuals tend to measure their interests as distinct—and often conflicting—with institutional interests	1 2 3 4 5	An environment in which institutional interests are defined to reflect individual interests and individuals view their interests as consistent with those of the institution

An Exercise for Organizational Assessment (continued)

An unstructured, individualistic approach to problem solving and decision making	1 2 3 4 5	A disciplined, predominantly participative approach to problem solving and decision making
An environment in which constant rework of tasks is accepted as the norm	1 2 3 4 5	An environment where task requirements are well defined and work is expected to be done right the first time. Constant striving for work improvement
A significantly internally competitive and parochial direction. A win/lose style	1 2 3 4 5	A cooperative overall company direction. A win/win style
An orientation to short-term objectives and actions with limited long-term perspective	1 2 3 4 5	The deliberate balances of long-term successes with short-term objectives
An environment in which there are no clear lines of authority that limit the decision-making process	1 2 3 4 5	An environment in which clear communication of the delegation of authority, responsibility, and accountability exists
A management style that tends to be remote and fault finding, and which instills a fear of failure	1 2 3 4 5	A participative and open management style that enables problems to be shared and solved cooperatively

Source: *Reprinted with permission from Strong Memorial Hospital at the University of Rochester, Rochester, NY, 1991.*

Figure 6.1. Assessing the hospital's culture and environment was a crucial step in deciding Strong's TQM strategy.

development of criteria and measures to monitor the success of their TQM efforts. Strong is the coordinating center of the Academic Medical Center Consortium (AMCC), a coalition of 12 top academic medical centers that conducts collaborative health services research.

The AMCC is working to develop the tools, techniques, and data systems that will help build the necessary infrastructure for maximally effective TQM. A common infrastructure will help each of the 12 hospitals in the consortium apply continuous quality improvement to clinical processes. Part of this infrastructure effort is the development of a common data base that will provide feedback on patient functional status and outcomes across the 12 hospitals. A combined data base of uniform hospital discharge data will be created during 1991 with pilot efforts to collect a common set of patient outcome data in 1992. While AMCC members vary in their implementation of formal TQM, they are all working to implement continuous quality improvement. See "Benchmarking" for more.

Brideau feels academic medical centers where research and education are combined with patient care present a fertile environment for TQM. The problem-solving process parallels the diagnostic and therapeutic approach taught to medical students and the scientific method of hypothesis testing that staff use as researchers. The OCPE has been a major catalyst in achieving Strong's vision of using research as a springboard to TQM. In 1987 Strong reorganized and expanded its clinical practice analysis activities and established the OCPE. Panzer and his staff provide guidance and support for research and improvement efforts throughout the hospital. Approximately 20% of the department's activities are devoted to the IPC program. Staff also provide analytical support for TQM activities, analyze QA data, support and coordinate AMCC-related activities, work with clinical department liaisons to review aggregate resource utilization, and support the hospital's grant research. At the same time research is promoting TQM, management believe TQM concepts and tools will also help improve research endeavors at Strong.

The emphasis on research at Strong is getting more staff involved in quality improvement. Nurses are one group whose jobs have been affected by the emphasis. Many have become heavily involved in IPC efforts, including a project that has evaluated a case management nursing care delivery system and its effects on costs and selected nurse and patient outcomes. The revamping of the hospital's system for professional advancement in nursing included a focus of incorporating more research into nursing.

Since senior management decided to train staff in family groups (see "Education"), Brideau foresaw the potential for staff to become frustrated. Beyond the initial project teams, senior managers have only been able to use the tools and techniques among themselves since other staff have not yet been trained. While TQM activities will begin at the department level once the department heads are trained, Brideau has told senior management to "be opportunistic in applying TQM methods" until then. For example, Roger J. Frankel, director for patient support services, inserts TQM into day-to-day management without actually calling it TQM. Staff are using TQM tools, such as brainstorming, in staff meetings without even knowing it. "These meetings help build bridges between management and staff and help foster the team approach," Frankel says. Susan Powell, director of clinical support services, plays the unofficial facilitator with staff, leading them through problem solving with a series of questions. For example, when staff in phlebotomy services saw an increase in STAT requests for inpatient blood samples, they looked into the causes for the increase and came up with solutions.

QI Process

Strong has adopted Xerox's six-step approach to problem solving illustrated in Figure 6.2 (page 178). As the figure illustrates, Xerox's model provides two approaches—one for problem-solving, which staff use when trying to improve an existing process, and one for quality improvement, which staff use for new process design or for major restructuring of processes. The case study (page 182) illustrates how the preoperative testing team used the problem-solving approach.

As discussed in "History," a Quality Resource Group, composed of a core group of hospital employees and physicians, supports team efforts through their combined roles as facilitators, trainers, and consultants.

As Table 6.1 (page 179) illustrates, the steps involved in completing an IPC research project are similar to the problem-solving steps Strong's quality improvement teams go through to investigate administrative or support processes. The similarity helps staff see research as a springboard into TQM. Table 6.2 (pages 180–181) provides a list of many of the IPC projects and quality improvement teams underway at Strong. Each year, approximately 30 requests for proposals are submitted for IPC grants. Physician researchers, initially Patricia Franklin, MD, and Edgar Black, MD, have overseen program operations. Based on their institutional importance relative to cost and quality, feasibility, and scientific validity, an average of ten research projects are

Problem-Solving and Quality Improvement Processsess

PSP Steps of Problem Solving		QIP Steps of Quality Improvement
Diagnostic Journey: 1. Define the problem cause 2. Determine root cause	Plan	1. Identify output 2. Identify customer 3. Identify customer requirements 4. Translate requirements into supplier specifications
Remedial Journey: 3. Generate potential solutions 4. Select and plan solution 5. Implement solution		5. Identify steps in work process 6. Select measurements 7. Determine process capability
	Do	8. Produce output
Check Performance:	Check	9. Evaluate results
6. Evaluate solution	Act	10. Recycle

Source: These processes were developed by Xerox Corporation, Rochester, NY, as the foundation of its Leadership Through Quality corporatewide management process. Reprinted with permission.

Figure 6.2. The Xerox problem-solving method that Strong adapted provides two approaches—one for problem solving and one for quality improvement.

awarded; these are grants between $5,000 and $20,000 each.

QA/QI Relationship

Brideau sees QA as an integral element of TQM. Presently, QA activities are being conducted side by side with TQM efforts at Strong. Jeanne Dent, director quality management, is investigating how QA information can be used in TQM activities that focus on processes and systems. QA staff are members of the Quality Resource Group that supports TQM.

Education

Strong has adopted Xerox's group approach to training. Staff receive intensive TQM education in peer or family groups. For example, all senior management completed their TQM training together. Beginning in the fall of 1991, all department managers and chiefs of clinical

Table 6.1. Comparison Between Research Approach and Xerox's Problem-Solving Model

IPC Problem-Solving Approach	Xerox's Problem-Solving Model
Issue request for proposal with priority areas listed. Clinicians and researchers propose study ideas	List and prioritize process or problems*
Full proposal submitted by team of researchers	Define project and team*
Research proposal defines study subjects, methods, and staff. Review panel and hospital leadership select studies to be funded. Plans for project defined prior to final approval	Define the problem cause
Project begins patient recruitment and data collection. Data analyzed	Determine the root cause
Results identify possible implementation mechanisms	Generate potential solutions
Implement design	Select and plan solution
Implement	Implement solution
Follow up data collected	Evaluate solution
Analyze and determine next steps	Begin cycle again as needed

These steps are not included in Figure 6.2 but usually occur during problem solving.

Source: *Developed by Robert Panzer, MD; Leo Brideau; and Jeanne Dent, Strong Memorial Hospital , University of Rochester, Rochester, NY, 1991. Reprinted with permission.*

services, together with their program management teams, will undergo 34 hours of training over a ten-week period. Every two weeks, all 150 managers and clinical chiefs will spend a half day together in training. In the spring and fall of 1992, the remaining 270 supervisors will be trained. Eventually line staff will be trained and department

Table 6.2. A Sample of Strong's Team Activities and IPC Projects

Team Activities

Improving the research process (OCPE Project). This project focused on ways to decrease delays in the research process, improve project documentation, decrease variability in the conduct of particular phases of research projects, and improve knowledge of the research process among staff members who execute research projects. Project planning, tracking, and summary documents were developed to improve documentation of research projects and to provide guidance for staff on the conduct of all phases of research projects. The *Research Reference Manual*, which describes all the processes involved in conducting each phase of a research project, was also developed.

Meeting information needs (OCPE Project). This project studied the process of responding to requests for clinical information (for example, providing length of stay or mortality information to Strong physicians and administrators). Two techniques for improving OCPE's reporting services were implemented: a revised data dictionary that is continuously reviewed and updated and a technical support network composed of experienced staff to assist and tutor other staff in the use of computer hardware and software maintained in the office.

Innovations in Patient Care

Focused discharge planning with adult medicine patients. This prospective study was designed to reduce the length of stay in elderly medicine patients through the early assessment of their discharge needs by community health nurses in addition to social work staff. The study indicated that an average stay of 1 ½ days was reduced in the study population. As a result of these findings, community health nurses were hired to screen all medicine patients 65 years and older. The study was expanded to orthopaedics and general surgery units.

Comparison of heparinized saline and normal saline in heparin locks in children. This study was a randomized, double-blind trial conducted to determine if duration of intermittent access, intravenous-line patency was different when pediatric patients receive a normal saline flush, rather than a heparinized saline flush. The study found no significant difference in the number of hours the line remained on the patient. Line longevity was positively correlated with the number of times the line was used, suggesting that the process of flushing is more important than is the agent used to flush. Normal saline became standard practice, which increased efficiency and reduced cost.

Serial work-up of cerebrospinal fluid analysis in children with possible meningitis. This study was conducted to test the hypothesis that a normal cell count and negative Gram stain on cerebrospinal fluid (CSF) analysis in children younger than three years is a sensitive screen

---

**Table 6.2. A Sample of Strong's Team Activities
and IPC Projects (continued)**

for meningitis and would generally eliminate the need for further CSF testing (CSF, glucose, protein, or differential). The hypothesis was supported by the study data, and a new laboratory order form is being designed to implement the change. This should result in reduced costs while maintaining high-quality care.

Fever detection study: Vital sign measurements combined with clinical assessment to detect fever in pediatric patients. This study was a prospective, randomized clinical trial conducted to determine if a schedule of reduced frequency vital sign measurement, combined with nurse clinical judgements, can detect as many fevers in hospitalized children as high frequency vital sign assessment. The hypothesis was supported, and the change in clinical practice became standard care.

---

managers and the clinical chiefs will begin a project with their staff using TQM concepts, just as the Steering Committee began TQM projects after training. The project teams created at the end of training will be built around the "family groups" that went through training together, and will take on process improvement projects in their area of common interest.

The hospital selected RIT to help provide training "in large part because of their knowledge of the Xerox experience," Brideau says. The University of Rochester, of which Strong is a component, is a national leader in a number of areas, but not TQM education. However, following the "train-the-trainer" approach, senior management and the Quality Resource Group are slowly assuming all training responsibilities. For example, while senior management and the Quality Resource Group are trained by RIT, they will help train department managers and clinical chiefs. The Quality Resource Group is developing training materials specific to Strong for this purpose. The first group of facilitators were also trained by RIT, but these facilitators in turn are developing their own facilitators' manual for the Quality Resource Group to use when training the next group of facilitators. Further, the hospital has developed its own training manual.

Brideau advises considering how a hospital is organized (that is, by department, by program) when deciding on a training approach. He feels Strong made the correct choice to train horizontally across

(continued on page 188)

181

Case Study
The Story of Strong's Preoperative Test Result Quality Improvement Project

Background

During the summer of 1989 an anesthesiologist and orthopaedic surgeon expressed their concerns to the Quality Assurance Committee that electrocardiogram (EKG) reports and laboratory reports were frequently missing from the patients' record at the time of surgery. This incomplete medical record could result in the following:

- Delay or rescheduling of surgery, resulting in inefficient use of the operating room;
- Less optimal patient care;
- Poor customer relations (both patient and physician dissatisfaction); and
- Revenue loss for hospital and physician.

The chief operating officer of Strong recommended that a quality improvement team be created to analyze the problem and implement solutions. A team composed of all stakeholders was assembled in September 1989 (see Table 6.A, page 183), and a problem statement developed (see Table 6.B, page 184). Once underway, the project team went through three phases of problem solving: diagnostic, remedial, and monitoring.

Diagnostic Phase

The diagnostic phase sought to identify the major aspects of the problem through the use of several quality improvement (QI) tools. First, baseline data collection by anesthesiologists in the operating room more clearly defined the extent of the problem (see Figure 6.A, page 185). Next a flowchart was developed, which followed the preoperative test ordering process from physician referral to the patient's admission for surgery. All functions involved in the process became a part of the flowchart. These included the admitting office, heart station, laboratory medicine, and medical records components. A cause-and-effect diagram was also constructed by team members in order to identify all possible causes of the problem (see Figure 6.B, page 186).

A Pareto chart, based on heart station data collection, was then created to identify the extent to which the various causes contributed to the problem (see Figure 6.C, page 187). Additional data collection was conducted to determine if physicians followed hospital protocol for ordering preoperative tests.

The use of quality improvement tools outlined above revealed the

Table 6.A. Preoperative Test Results Quality Improvement Project Team Members

Vivian Palladoro, MS—Team Leader
Administrator, Laboratory Medicine

Jeanne N. Dent—Facilitator
Associate Director for Quality Improvement

Laurie A. Barton
Assistant, Quality Assurance Coordinator

Alice B. Basford, MD
Clinical Associate Professor, Anesthesiology

Laura L. Butler
Supervisor, Heart Station

Diane S. Clement, RN
Quality Assurance Coordinator, Orthopaedics

Denni O. Day
Director, Operations Improvement

Darby B. Leyden, RN
Associate Clinical Chief, Surgical Nursing

Judy McMaster
Administrator, Medicine

Marilyn Morrealle
Supervisor, Medical Records

Vincent D. Pellegrini, Jr, MD
Assistant Professor, Orthopaedics

Melinda Spry
Assistant Quality Assurance Coordinator

David Strong
Director, Surgical Support Services

Deborah Tuttle
Associate Director of the Office of Clinical Practice Evaluation

Delores Wachtman
Manager, Patient Admission Services

---

following problems resulting in missing preoperative test results at the time of surgery:

1. The heart station did not always know that a patient was preoperative and did not consider EKG interpretation a top priority.

2. A telephone survey of a random sample of referring physicians demonstrated that physicians do not comply with the hospital's protocol for ordering preoperative tests.

3. A cardiology resident/fellow/faculty is not always readily available to interpret STAT EKGs.

4. House officers and nurses do not follow the heart station's service guidelines for deadlines and hours of operation.

5. The preoperative test completion for patients is not checked until late evening the night before surgery or early morning the day of surgery. This leads to STAT EKG requests on the day of surgery, often delaying surgery.

6. The patient's units are not receiving the operating room schedule for the next day in a timely fashion, resulting in delayed information to patient care units.

Additional problems encountered involved confusion regarding terminology, ineffective filing systems, use of incorrect requisitions, and untimely transfer of medical records from the emergency department to the patient care unit.

Remedial Phase
The following solutions were implemented as a result of diagnostic phase activities:

1. The EKG requisition was revised to include a preoperative designation box;

2. The committee has recommended that the hospital assign responsibility to a specific office for ongoing communication with physicians regarding policies and procedures;

Table 6.B. Problem Statement and Goal for Improvement

Problem statement. Twenty-four percent* of EKG results are not in the medical record at the time of surgery resulting in the increased incidence of STAT EKG requests for imminent elective surgery. Fourteen percent of CBC, Profile 6 and urinalysis results are not in the medical record at the time of surgery, resulting in the increased incidence of STAT laboratory requests for imminent elective surgery.

Goal for improvement statement. Design and implement a system that will result in 95% inclusion in the medical record of specific ordered preoperative exams (CBC, Profile 6, Urinalysis, and EKG) for adult elective surgical cases according to Strong's admission testing protocol.

* *January 1990 data collection.*

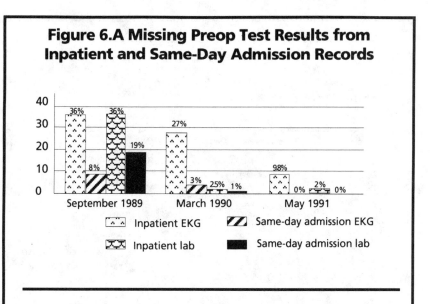

Figure 6.A Missing Preop Test Results from Inpatient and Same-Day Admission Records

3. The heart station medical director recommended, after a study to assess their interpretation accuracy, that third-year medical residents be allowed to provide final EKG interpretations when attending cardiologists are unavailable;

4. A letter was sent to house officers and an in-service program was conducted for nurses describing hours of service and heart station protocols for various tests;

5. The committee recommended that the feasibility of interfacing the operating room computer and the heart station computer be investigated to better identify surgical patients;

6. Nurses are now confirming the completion of preoperative tests for patients on the day prior to surgery rather than the night before or morning of surgery; and

7. The distribution list and delivery time of the operating room schedule is being revised and improved by the Operating Room Operations Committee.

In addition to the above-stated remedies, the committee members' standardized terms, conducted in-service sessions for secretaries and nurses, and modified medical records processing so that patient records were available to the patient care units on a timely basis.

Results

Data collection in May 1991 revealed that only 2% of lab results and 9.8% of EKG results were missing from the medical record at the time of surgery. The project team members were pleased to have imple-

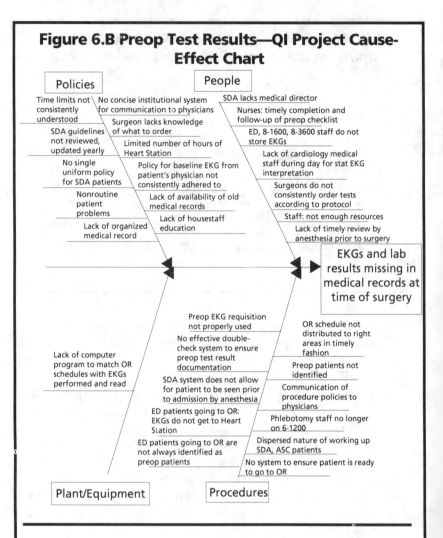

Figure 6.B Preop Test Results—QI Project Cause-Effect Chart

Policies

Time limits not consistently understood

No concise institutional system for communication to physicians

Surgeon lacks knowledge of what to order

SDA guidelines not reviewed, updated yearly

Limited number of hours of Heart Station

No single uniform policy for SDA patients

Policy for baseline EKG from patient's physician not consistently adhered to

Nonroutine patient problems

Lack of availability of old medical records

Lack of organized medical record

Lack of housestaff education

People

SDA lacks medical director

Nurses: timely completion and follow-up of preop checklist

ED, 8-1600, 8-3600 staff do not store EKGs

Lack of cardiology medical staff during day for stat EKG interpretation

Surgeons do not consistently order tests according to protocol

Staff: not enough resources

Lack of timely review by anesthesia prior to surgery

EKGs and lab results missing in medical records at time of surgery

Lack of computer program to match OR schedules with EKGs performed and read

Preop EKG requisition not properly used

No effective double-check system to ensure preop test result documentation

SDA system does not allow for patient to be seen prior to admission by anesthesia

ED patients going to OR: EKGs do not get to Heart Station

ED patients going to OR are not always identified as preop patients

OR schedule not distributed to right areas in timely fashion

Preop patients not identified

Communication of procedure policies to physicians

Phlebotomy staff no longer on 6-1200

Dispersed nature of working up SDA, ASC patients

No system to ensure patient is ready to go to OR

Plant/Equipment

Procedures

mented solutions at nominal cost that resulted in significant improvements in preoperative test ordering and reporting process.

Monitoring

The third phase of the project—monitoring—has been ongoing since initial solutions were implemented and quality assurance staff collected data (medical record checks in operating room) to determine the effectiveness of those solutions implemented. Data collection was then repeated periodically throughout the project in order to monitor the team's progress. With the goal for improvement at hand, plans are to continue ongoing monitoring under the direction of operating room

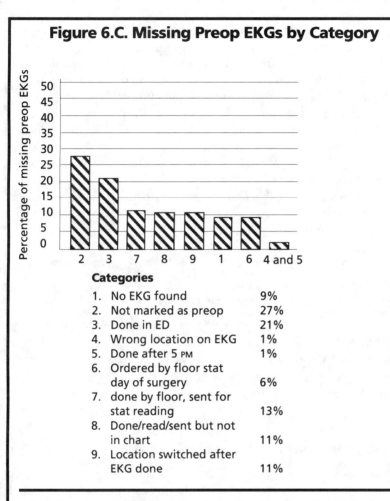

Figure 6.C. Missing Preop EKGs by Category

Categories

1.	No EKG found	9%
2.	Not marked as preop	27%
3.	Done in ED	21%
4.	Wrong location on EKG	1%
5.	Done after 5 PM	1%
6.	Ordered by floor stat day of surgery	6%
7.	done by floor, sent for stat reading	13%
8.	Done/read/sent but not in chart	11%
9.	Location switched after EKG done	11%

administration. A control chart will be developed and if the limits are exceeded, a team will form to initiate a problem-solving process.

Lessons Learned

In addition to the improvements made to the preoperative test result process, the team's experiences were valuable for the following lessons learned:

- Initial projects should have limited scope;
- All members of a project team should receive basic TQM training;
- A team leader and facilitator should have training in TQM concepts and methodologies, particularly team-building skills;
- The reward and recognition component is important, even at pilot team stage;

- Boundaries should be established for the project and the team should stay focused on its goal for improvement. Agree to refer certain tasks to other committees or teams (for example, the distribution problem of operating room schedules was referred to the Operating Room Operations Committee).
- Realize how dynamic the institution is. In the preoperative team's case, this required continuous checking (for example, a new computer system was installed during this project, the same-day admission center process changed, anesthesia appointed a new director of clinical affairs); and
- Know in advance that patience and an open mind are important attributes of all project team members—mistakes made become *invaluable* lessons learned.

Source: Developed and written by Vivian A. Palladoro, MS, Administrator Laboratory Medicine, and Jeanne N. Dent, RN, BSN, CPQA, Associate Director Quality Improvement, Strong Memorial Hospital, University of Rochester Medical Center, Rochester, NY, 1991. For more information, contact either Vivian A. Palladoro at 716/275-5129 or Jeanne N. Dent at 716/275-5205.

(continued from page 181)

disciplines since the hospital is organized in a matrix fashion. Brideau cautions that training vertically by department might send the wrong message. "Horizontal instruction allows people to talk to each other across disciplines," he says.

QI Supports

Customer feedback mechanisms. Strong has identified four major direct customer groups: patients and their families and friends, physicians and dentists who admit and care for patients at Strong, health care providers who refer patients, and employees and volunteers. Staff are seeking feedback from each of these groups in different ways. The patient relations department distributes a survey to patients when they are discharged. Approximately 85% of patients receive surveys, with an estimated 20%-25% response rate. Survey results are used to set goals for improvement as well as evaluate trends, according to Diane Healy, patient relations coordinator. Responses can be broken down by patient units and support units (for example, housekeeping) and trended over time. Departments often incorporate survey data into their QA activities, Healy says. Many departments perform their own surveys that complement the main survey. Healy provides quarterly analysis reports on patient feedback for management and includes them in her QA report. The office of planning and marketing has conducted a survey of referring physicians and is establishing a quick phone line for physicians to register their complaints. Some employee surveys are also being conducted through the human resources committee.

Reward and recognition. Staff are working to incorporate TQM concepts into Strong's performance review system. The Strong Quality Implementation Team will establish reward and recognition objectives and guidelines. Each level of management is expected to develop performance criteria regarding quality management for all positions accountable to them. "If TQM is not tied into the evaluation process, the message is that TQM is not important," Powell says. She feels management needs to build in an expectation of staff to participate in TQM efforts.

Information management. One function of the OCPE is to provide data and research support for quality improvement initiatives, including IPC projects. OCPE maintains a data base that meets the needs of physicians and administration, develops report packages that meet Joint Commission and regulator requirements, and provides information that encourages staff to participate in QA and utilization review. Deborah Tuttle, associate director, and Gary Katsanis, data administrator, explain that OCPE does more than simply provide data to staff; OCPE also assists in research and analysis. OCPE extracts data from the hospital information system using billing/discharge data and analyzes the data with a statistical analysis system. Staff restructure files and develop proxies for analysis. OCPE staff will also go out and collect data for studies when computerized information is not available, which is often the case in IPC studies. Clinical data collection is not centralized at Strong. Many departments collect their own data, and OCPE extracts the data as needed.

As part of the department's TQM initiatives, one team is working with its customers to make the data system more user friendly. According to Katsanis, his team has developed a data base dictionary and involved users in the data base conversion currently underway.

Supplier relationships. Strong treats its in-house suppliers as employees. For example, Ray Bucknell reports to Strong's department of materials management, although he is an employee of UARCO, a forms management company, and he attends department head meetings and is a member of the Medical Records Committee. Eventually, Strong envisions involving suppliers in team activities. Many suppliers, such as UARCO, are already implementing TQM and are excited about working with Strong in this manner.

Benchmarking. Strong belongs to a variety of consortiums, including the Premier Hospital Alliance, Inc, National Demonstration Project's Quality Management Network, and AMCC. Headquartered at the University of Rochester Medical Center, AMCC includes 12 other academic medical centers, including Johns Hopkins Medical Center, Massachusetts General Hospital, and the Mayo Clinic. The research that AMCC is conducting is intended to lead to the development of methods, criteria, and policy guidelines needed to improve health care outcomes. As discussed in "Strategy," members of AMCC are working on the creation of a common outcome management infrastructure and data system that will help all 12 hospitals apply continuous quality improvement.

Physician Involvement

Griner and Brideau emphasize that the administration of every institution must look at its relationship with the medical staff before beginning to approach physicians with TQM. The appropriate approach will be unique to different hospitals, they say. At Strong, senior management first won the support of the clinical chiefs of the hospital departments. Since they are the chairs of academic departments as well, their support was critical. At a 1 ½-day retreat, Griner, Brideau, Pittman, and Panzer presented the rationale for seeking to transform Strong into a "total quality" institution to the clinical chiefs. The reasons included quality for its own sake, reduced costs through improved quality, Strong's responsibility as a teaching hospital, and improved employee satisfaction. In addition, they cautioned that the high costs of Strong's services could place the hospital at a competitive disadvantage over the next several years, unless the incremental value of those higher costs could be conclusively demonstrated and continually enhanced. They demonstrated how TQM was the best way to handle this potential crisis. A videotape about paradigm shifts[7] was received enthusiastically. All chiefs have begun formal training as a group, and training will be provided to any other member of the medical staff who desires it.

Clinical chiefs at Strong emphasize several issues hospitals should consider when approaching physicians with TQM:

- Irwin N. Frank, MD, senior director and medical director, stressed that the broader aspects of TQM such as improved patient care and access should be emphasized as well as decreased costs. If physicians see TQM only as a way for the hospital to save money they won't buy in, he says. Senior management believe the success of the IPC program will help demonstrate the link between quality and costs. As discussed in "Philosophy," the IPC program has already begun to shift attitudes about the linkage.

- Dean Arvan, MD, director, laboratory medicine, says he is very impressed by the ideas of TQM but recognizes that TQM is going to "take considerable effort." Before physicians will buy in, he feels senior management will have to complete some demonstration projects. "They need to convince people that the outcome is worth the up-front effort," that it is worth the "amount of time necessary to become familiar with concepts."

- Raymond J. Mayewski, MD, associate chairman of clinical affairs in the department of medicine, also believes time is a major deterrent for physicians. He stresses that, until a cultural change has been achieved, staff will need some incentives to become involved in TQM. Pointing out that incentives do not necessarily have to be monetary, he suggests management might lure physicians by focusing on areas of particular interest to them.

As an academic medical center, resident physicians provide a large percentage of patient care at Strong. This presents a unique barrier to Strong's TQM rollout: How is quality emphasized within a learning environment? Strong is approaching this barrier in several ways. Senior management emphasize that services at Strong are provided by attending physicians and residents who work under their guidance. This allows the resident to learn from the attending physician by seeing quality service. Griner is also hoping to change the processes in which residents are involved by "making the right path the path of least resistance." By planning ahead and decreasing the complexity of the work residents have to accomplish, there is less possibility that mistakes and rework will occur. For example, residents used to calculate each baby's intravenous formula in the neonatal intensive care unit with hand calculators. To simplify the process, a computer program was designed to assist in the procedure. As a result, formula calculation time has been reduced from 20 minutes per baby to 2 minutes, and the number of resident errors were reduced from several per week to zero over a one-year period. Because of the demands on residents, it is difficult for them "to sit still for 36 hours of training or give time to teams," Brideau says. Eventually he hopes to have some didactic sessions for residents on TQM and to involve leaders such as chief residents in more formal training.

Conclusion

Strong is testing the boundaries of TQM application within the hospital environment, moving beyond the improvement of support or administrative processes to clinical process improvement. Brideau says it is too early to predict if Strong's approach will be one all other academic medical centers should pursue. With research and educational resources readily available, academic health centers are in a unique position to explore the depths of TQM application. The experiences of Strong will prove valuable to all hospitals making the transition to a TQM culture.

References

1. Brideau LP, et al: Innovations in clinical practice through hospital-funded grants. *Acad Med* pp 355–360, 1990.

2. Panzer RJ: Changing clinical practices through hospital-funded, small grants. *The Quality Letter.* Mar 1991, pp 6–9.

3. The Rochester experiment. *Financial World Magazine,* Jan 10, 1989.

4. Taylor P: *The Health Care System of Rochester, New York. Its History and Achievements.* Book released in conjunction with the 1991 annual meeting of Blue Cross and Blue Shield of the Rochester area, Feb 12, 1991.

5. Evans J: Blue Cross seeks increase. *Rochester Democrat & Chronicle.* Rochester, NY, Oct 2, 1990.

6. Greater Rochester Chamber of Commerce and Windsor Publications: *Rochester: An Imaging & Optics Capital of the World.* Rochester, NY.

7. Barker J: *Discovering the Future.* Burnsville, MN: Chart House International, 1989.

7 Shared Experiences

The six hospitals profiled in *Striving Toward Improvement* vary in size, location, mission, ownership, and organizational structure. They also use several different quality improvement (QI) models with distinct philosophies and areas of emphasis. Despite the differences among these organizations, they have had remarkably similar experiences that cover approaches to implementation, characteristics of a successful transition, and lessons learned. While every hospital did not identify each of the issues discussed in this chapter, the common characteristics were described by most of the hospitals. The following summary is not intended to imply that there is a single right way to implement QI, nor that the approaches are appropriate for all organizations. Rather, it is an attempt to share the experiences of the hospitals that have embarked upon the journey.

The Transition and the Role of Leaders

The chief executive officer usually served as the catalyst for change within the hospital. Leadership involvement, including senior management, board members, and physician, nurse, and other clinical leaders, was found to be critical for a successful transition. The first few years of the transition required considerable energy and time commitments from leaders. John Bingham at Magic Valley estimated he spends 50% of this time on QI activities, and Philip Newbold said that in the beginning of Memorial's efforts, he spent a minimum of two hours a day on QI. Now QI has been blended into his daily routine. Many agreed with Newbold and felt strongly that it has become (and should be) an integral part of daily work life that cannot be separately identified.

A steering committee or quality council, composed of senior management, provided general guidance and oversight in the transition. This group was usually equivalent to the regular management team, although in some cases there were variations in membership.

For example, Wright-Patterson has included their patient relations coordinator on the Quality Council, and Bethesda's Steering Committee includes several medical staff members. The creation of a quality council ensured leadership direction and active participation. It usually identified major areas of focus for QI efforts and guided and approved team activities. At Parkview, for example, the Quality Council chose five hospitalwide systems (for example, clinical results reporting) that have become a major QI focus for the entire organization. Many teams were created to focus on each of these five systems. The appointment of a QI "coach" to facilitate the efforts of the quality council was felt to be useful in the initial stages of the transition. The QI coach assists management with the transition in areas such as education, use of QI tools, and rollout within the organization. QI coaches frequently were members of the quality council.

Active support from the governing body early in the process was needed not only for approval of the new direction but also because of the magnitude of the change involved and because resource commitments must be made before results were realized. Supportive board members at these hospitals were frequently involved in QI in their own organizations. For example, Strong Memorial has a representative from Xerox, a recent Malcolm Baldrige award winner, on its board. Board members often participated in site visits made by leaders to other QI organizations both inside and outside health care. The hospital leaders found such visits useful in making the initial decision to move to QI and in determining which QI model to adopt.

Organizations adopted either an established approach to QI (for example, Deming, Juran) or developed their own unique model, which is often a hybrid of different approaches. For example, Parkview is devoted primarily to Deming's philosophy, while Memorial's model is based largely on Juran mixed with Deming's and Senge's concepts. The selection of a QI model was based on the organization's philosophical agreement with underlying concepts. Commitment to a single approach was usually made with the expectation that it would not be changed. The use of more than one model in an organization could lead to confusion concerning direction. The hospitals studied in this book stressed the importance of a common language within the organization that promotes cross-functional QI efforts, enhances consistency, and facilitates efforts to measure progress. This was felt to be best achieved by long-term commitment to a single model.

The six hospitals reported that in a QI environment, the roles of leaders and other managers changes from one of dictator, controller, and exhorter to champion, mentor, and coach. These leaders exhibited behaviors consistent with QI and demonstrated a commitment to its philosophy and methods, commonly referred to as "walking the talk." Most senior management actively participated in QI activities by undergoing extensive education, engaging in their own process improvement efforts, personally providing training to staff, and assigning specific senior management "sponsors" to teams. These leaders established direction, displayed "constancy of purpose," and provided continual guidance to encourage change in others. Sharon Fischer, QI coach at Magic Valley, sums up the initial attitude of many middle managers and staff at each of the six hospitals—"At first, most staff thought QI was another fad that would pass." It took constancy of purpose demonstrated by management to change their minds.

Although QI more actively engages staff in future planning, the transition was not an egalitarian process in these hospitals; the pursuit of QI was an explicit management decision. Leaders did not delegate overall responsibility for QI implementation—they assumed it themselves. They established a structure that included a formal problem-solving process, use of statistical methods and QI tools, reliance on data, training on the appropriate use of these tools, and rewards for success. This enabled staff to address issues in a more open and, therefore, productive manner and to take ownership of the structure provided to them. There appeared to be a direct relationship between the use of this structure and staff's demonstration of a sense of inquiry, pride in work, restlessness with the status quo, and confidence that they could use their talents to make effective changes. Rather than stifling staff, the formal structure provided by management led to their "liberation"—empowerment to investigate and improve those processes that affected them.

The hospitals found that organizationwide acceptance of QI concepts was necessary before extensive change could occur. An antecedent environment that has already embraced some of the philosophical underpinnings of QI often assisted in the transition. For example, Memorial has been focusing on customer needs and staff empowerment, Bethesda has placed strong reliance on data for decision making, and Wright-Patterson and Strong have moved to matrix management at the department level, which has helped emphasize collaboration between disciplines.

Results did not appear overnight; the hospitals measure the transition time in years. Early successes were critical to maintaining enthusiasm, and leaders often ensured that such successes were achieved through the careful selection of QI projects and the provision of support and resources.

Vision

A written vision statement that broadly describes future goals of the organization was usually developed early on to focus QI efforts. The vision statement was typically developed by senior management, although in several cases the governing body actively participated. The hospitals believed that the vision must be regularly communicated to staff in order to obtain support for the transition. Different methods have been used to communicate this vision. Wright-Patterson, for example, has displayed its mission and vision on bulletin boards across the medical center and distributed a brochure outlining its QI philosophy to all staff, patients, and visitors. Several of the hospitals are also asking each department to develop a departmental vision that aligns with the hospital vision. Most organizations learned that, unless there is a shared vision and widespread acceptance of QI principles, success is more difficult to achieve.

The long-term goal for the six hospitals studied is a totally transformed organization. The leaders believe that it is not enough to be satisfied with incremental improvements in existing functions. In several hospitals, vision statements reflected this organizational transformation. Many hospitals developed measures of success to help them assess progress in reaching this desired future state. For example, senior management at Parkview developed measurements to assess key quality characteristics of the future of the hospital. In several cases, the vision was used to set boundaries for QI activities and teams engaged in projects that contributed to the achievement of the vision.

Some, such as Magic Valley, used QI as an opportunity to expand their vision beyond the walls of the hospital into the community, establishing partnerships between the hospital and those they serve.

Strategy and Rollout

While the decision to pursue QI may be due to an impending organizational crisis, it was more often the result of philosophical agreement with the concepts in the six hospitals. However, many viewed QI as providing the necessary tools to carry an organization through a crisis or to overcome negative environmental forces.

QI became an integral part of regular business strategies, and customer feedback was often an important component of strategic planning. Most, in retrospect, would have concentrated more on planning early in the process, and some had to backtrack to focus on planning. Typical to the experience of many of the hospitals, Strong formed several teams at the beginning of its QI efforts; however, because there was not a core understanding of QI goals throughout the hospital, these teams had to work in relative isolation. Now Strong is concentrating more on planning than a rapid expansion of teams. In addition, many cautioned that the QI expectations within the plan should not exceed the organization's ability to achieve them. It was suggested that planning be structured so it is consistent with the progression of staff training in such areas as quality awareness, organization vision, and process improvement.

Hospitals have found that successful implementation always takes longer than expected and a lull frequently seems to occur somewhere in the process. The lull was frequently attributed to overtraining, insufficient direction, or simply a normal waning of initial enthusiasm. Continued management commitment and, in some cases, special efforts were required to regain momentum.

QI in these hospitals was not synonymous with chartered team activities. For example, individual departments frequently were required to initiate their own QI activities, including the identification of internal customers and suppliers, development of quality plans, and intradepartmental process improvement activities. The development of an implementation or rollout plan for the hospital (including departmental priorities linked to hospital goals) usually supported the application and integration of QI principles and methods into the daily operations of the hospital. Departments typically needed management assistance early in the process with the identification of internal customers and other quality planning efforts. These department efforts involved all staff and, sometimes because of this, middle management felt threatened by a perceived loss of control or power, leading to some degree of resistance at this level. As key participants in important hospital processes, nurses were usually enthusiastically involved in QI efforts. The recent movement in nursing toward empowerment was seen as consistent with and useful in QI. For example, Magic Valley and Strong are adopting clinical practice nursing models that will result in greater decentralization and shared governance. At Memorial, which has been involved in empowerment and shared governance for several years, nurses have often taken the lead in department and organizationwide QI activities.

Consultants were helpful in developing rollout plans and educational materials. However, many hospitals cautioned that careful selection of the appropriate consultant and ensuring that the consultant's approach meets the unique needs of the organization is critical. Early implementation efforts can be derailed by attempting to adopt a boilerplate that is not relevant to the organization.

Quality assurance (QA) and QI were usually separate functions, particularly in the initial stages. Many hospitals felt it was important to take the time to understand how QA requirements can be met in the context of QI. The chapters on Wright-Patterson, Memorial, and Magic Valley describe approaches to this issue. Most plan to integrate these functions in the future. Several indicated that QA would become a component of QI in the future as well as a source for issues to address through the QI process.

QI Teams

Several hospitals initiated QI efforts with pilot teams to assess how well the process would work within the organization and/or to demonstrate the effectiveness of QI methods. These pilot efforts led to improvements in team functions, such as implementing just-in-time training on tools and assigning a management sponsor to teams.

Teams tended to focus more on administrative processes than clinical issues in the initial stages of the transition because organizations felt it would be easier to achieve initial success in these areas. Several hospitals, however, have begun to explore clinical issues. Bethesda is well on its way, exploring the treatment of asthma patients, cesarean sections and hip replacements, and Wright-Patterson has a team exploring the diagnostic process for potential breast cancer, from ordering mammograms to surgery. A few hospitals, including Memorial and Strong, are using critical paths to apply QI in clinical areas.

Most organizations found that initial team projects should be carefully selected by management because hospitals encountered problems when all proposed teams were allowed to form on their own initiative. Memorial refers to these as "skunk teams." In several instances, management was unable to provide the needed resources to teams (education, facilitators) or support the implementation of proposed solutions. In addition, management wanted to focus efforts on organizational priorities and wanted to ensure that teams did not conflict with macro processes. As a result, QI teams were typically chartered by the Quality Council to focus on areas identified as important to the hospital and recommendations were usually brought to the Council for approval. A structured chartering process was usually followed.

Nevertheless, unchartered teams were initiated by staff in some hospitals to explore issues within their areas of responsibility. Unchartered teams usually addressed intradepartmental issues or those that were limited in scope. Several hospitals expected that the number of such teams would increase as staff became more experienced with QI concepts and methods.

Teams needed the support of trained facilitators with QI methods and tools, particularly in the early stages of implementation. Most hospitals learned that the number of teams should be limited to the number of facilitators available because teams frequently became ineffective if they operated without facilitator guidance. Bethesda, Memorial, Parkview, and others are training additional facilitators to keep up with the demand for teams. Hospitals learned that issues addressed by teams should be narrowly focused; teams often developed charters that were too broad and as a result floundered. At Bethesda, the registration team, which was asked to investigate alternatives to or make improvements in the entire registration process, ended up focusing on outpatient registration after data showed that was where the heaviest volume occurred.

A structured process improvement method was used by each of the hospitals profiled and was applied to team efforts, in interdepartmental or intradepartmental QI efforts, and in daily activities. These methods often varied in the number of steps involved: FOCUS-PDCA has 9 steps and is used by Parkview, Magic Valley, and Wright-Patterson; Bethesda's approach has 13 steps; Strong's has 6; and Memorial's has 7. But all contained similar basic elements, such as identifying the issue, collecting data for issue clarification, identifying solutions, selecting a pilot solution, testing the solution, implementing the change, and monitoring to maintain the gain.

Internal communication was considered important for creating a common understanding and language within the organization, and for enhancing awareness of QI activities. Storyboards, storybooks, newsletters, and forums were found to be very effective in fostering such communication.

Education

All six hospitals earmarked significant financial and human resources for training all staff in QI concepts and tools. Some even identified resources for service coverage while staff were being trained.

In many cases, senior management attended external seminars for initial QI education. Most hospitals determined, however, that it would be too costly to rely on external resources for general staff education, and training materials were either developed or adapted internally to meet the unique needs of the hospital. For example, Bethesda developed an awareness course that used specific QI examples from their hospital. Many different educational vehicles were made available to staff, including courses, audio-visual materials, books and articles, journal clubs, and forums.

Training usually began at the top and was cascaded down through the organization. QI was introduced to new staff in orientation training. Typically, senior management actively participated in staff training by teaching courses.

Most organizations found it counterproductive to provide too much training at once. In the beginning, structures that allowed staff to apply new knowledge (such as functioning teams or formal departmental QI activities) were usually not in place. This is a situation Philip Newbold at Memorial referred to as "dressing everyone up for the dance with no dance to go to." In some cases, this led to frustration and a lack of future support for QI efforts. Through experience, hospitals found that the most effective approach was to provide general QI awareness training to staff followed by just-in-time training to teams and departments on QI tools as needed.

Physician Involvement

Some hospitals delayed active physician involvement in QI until the effectiveness of the methods was demonstrated and to assure that the organization could support their participation. In addition, time requirements for up front training and team participation was recognized as a barrier to physician involvement. Several hospitals identified ways to incrementally involve physicians in QI before formal introduction to the medical staff. Bethesda decided to involve physicians initially as consultants to teams addressing administrative issues rather than full members. In several cases, physicians participated on teams addressing administrative issues in areas of interest to them,

such as waiting times in the operating room or emergency department; improvements in these areas demonstrated the value of QI
methods to physicians. Both Magic Valley and Bethesda encouraged
physicians to become involved in QI projects in their own offices.

In many cases, a physician was hired to assist with the rollout of QI
within the medical staff. Initial physician involvement was also accomplished by identifying interested individuals to serve as champions for other physicians. Both approaches provided role models to
encourage more widespread physician involvement. Physician interest was often enhanced when they realized QI can focus on problems
relevant to them, such as variation in medical practice. They also have
been intrigued by the focus on systems improvement rather than
individuals (bad apples), and because QI is a scientific process using
sound data, QI has also helped physicians understand how they fit into
the customer-supplier chain within the hospital.

The language of QI may be foreign to physicians initially. Several
hospitals have developed special training methods that translate these
concepts into familiar terms and meet other unique needs of physicians.

QI Supports

Most hospitals identified a variety of internal and external customers
that included patients, families, employers, payers, and the general
community. Regular feedback (with some variation in frequency) was
gathered from identified customers, and this information was incorporated into QI efforts. Wright-Patterson, for example, identified that
access to the hospital was the major concern of patients and directed
QI efforts to that area. A number of techniques were used to obtain
customer input, including surveys, telephone interviews, and focus
groups; several hospitals combined techniques. For example, Bethesda
held a focus group with physicians to gather qualitative data and
subsequently conducted a telephone survey to a larger sample to
gather quantitative data. Organizations used outside consultants,
internal resources, or a combination of both to collect customer
information. Hospitals were also making efforts to refine and increase
the sophistication of data collection instruments and to reduce the
possibility of biased data.

Quality relationships with suppliers were beginning to be established
by hospitals. Although generally not yet widespread, these relationships
involved contractual agreements, informal efforts to resolve specific

issues, or supplier participation on QI teams. Memorial has an organ procurement team that involves representatives from two organ banks and Johnson & Johnson has a representative on Bethesda's wound closure team. Most expected such arrangements to increase in the future and that supplier selection would be based as much on quality as cost.

All the hospitals profiled in this book engaged in some form of benchmarking. This involved participating in comparative data bases, visiting other QI organizations, and studying methods that others use for specific processes to identify opportunities for improvement. Examples of the latter included billing processes, performance feedback/reward systems, and customer/guest relations. Benchmarking activities were conducted both within the health care field and with outside manufacturing and service industries.

The sophistication of information services and the ability to provide computer support for QI activities varied among the hospitals. Even in those hospitals with the most sophisticated computer systems, the data needed by teams were often not readily available in existing data bases. As a result, much information was collected manually or special programs were written to assist with data collection and analysis. Most organizations noted that there was a need for a greater integration of data systems to support QI efforts and increased staff access to data. A need for more process data was also noted.* Many hospitals recognized that additional financial resources may be required to support data collection, as well as for assessing customer needs, educational efforts, and consultants.

A number of these hospitals were reexamining traditional performance evaluation processes and personnel policies in the context of QI philosophy. As described in the earlier chapters, hospitals were experimenting with the elimination of traditional merit systems, introduction of "gain sharing" programs, and redesign of performance feedback mechanisms. There was some concern about striking the proper balance between recognition of group efforts and rewarding outstanding individual performance, and most agreed that the ultimate solution is yet to be found. Other forms of reward and recognition being used included individual team recognition and quality celebrations.

---

* Sue Weinstein at Bethesda provided the following example of process versus outcome data related to wound homeostasis: an outcome datum is the length of time a wound bled while a process datum is the length of time the wound was compressed.

8 A Roundtable Discussion on QI Issues

After each hospital was visited, the leaders of all six hospitals were brought together for a roundtable discussion of issues that arose during the site visits. The issues discussed fell under seven topics: leadership, implementing quality improvement (QI), barriers/resistance, medical staff involvement, cultural change, institutionalizing QI, and external environment. The following is a transcript of that discussion.

PARTICIPANTS

John Anderson, MD, JD Commander	USAF Medical Center, Wright-Patterson
John Bingham Administrator	Magic Valley Regional Medical Center
Paul Griner, MD General Director	Strong Memorial Hospital of the University of Rochester
Robert Panzer, MD* Director of Clinical Practice Evaluation	Strong Memorial Hospital of the University of Rochester
Philip Newbold President and Chief Executive Officer	Memorial Hospital and Health System
Michael Pugh President and Chief Executive Officer	Parkview Episcopal Medical Center
L. Thomas Wilburn Chairman, President, and Chief Executive Officer	Bethesda Hospital, Inc

FACILITATOR

James A. Prevost, MD Director, Applications Research	Joint Commission on Accreditation of Healthcare Organizations

---

*Paul Griner, MD, was unable to stay for the entire discussion. Bob Panzer, MD, represented Strong Memorial Hospital after Dr Griner left.

LEADERSHIP

Prevost: I had the opportunity to interview each of you on the subject of leadership during the site visit to your hospital. All the interviews began with the same question: What are the most important characteristics of a chief executive officer and leader in a hospital adopting quality improvement (QI)?* After we completed all the site visits, we found that many of the characteristics noted by each of you were, in fact, shared by all of you.

First, you all said the chief executive officer must demonstrate leadership by having, promoting, and articulating a QI vision for the hospital. This vision is a transforming cause in which hospital staff can identify their own individual dreams and goals within the vision.

Second, chief executive officers must be good communicators.

Third, you must have teaching skills and yourselves be learners.

Fourth, chief executive officers in QI hospitals must possess a restlessness with the status quo. You cannot be maintenance managers. Improving the hospital culture in support of patient care is always on your minds.

Fifth, chief executive officers should have a fundamental belief in the worth of people. That's how Phil Newbold put it. Tom Wilburn talked about respect. John Bingham talked about passion, love. John Anderson mentioned trust. This belief includes a respect for those people closest to

the work—that they know best how to improve their work. This belief keeps the hospital leader from jumping in with the solution without first involving others and from undermining the problem-solving process.

The sixth characteristic is a capacity to tolerate change and the chaos that goes with it.

The seventh is high energy and the willingness to take the time to carry on the QI effort over the long run.

Again, all of you mentioned these seven characteristics, possibly with a different emphasis or meaning. So, let's begin. What are your comments about these seven characteristics? Are there other characteristics? What are the features of a leader and chief executive officer in a QI hospital?

Griner: One element of leadership necessary for the success of total quality management (TQM) is a basic understanding that the most important TQM principles are independent of the specific methods that each of us, as hospital leaders, are applying. Methodology is less important than the leader's ability to articulate those TQM principles to staff. For instance, the leader's inability to tolerate systems problems or restlessness with the status quo, the ability to give constant attention to improving services, the importance placed on the use of data to support problem solving and change, the ability to communicate the essential understanding that as professionals

---

* *The acronyms QI (quality improvement), TQM (total quality management), and CQI (continuous quality improvement) are used interchangeably throughout the roundtable discussion to refer to the quality efforts the six hospitals are instituting. In the discussion of particular hospitals, the term used is that employed by the hospital.*

it is our responsibility to evaluate ourselves constantly, and the focus on customers—all of these, to me, are critical elements in continuous quality improvement (CQI) that are independent of the methods leaders apply.

There's an important credibility issue in promoting principles rather than methods, particularly for the nonbelievers. It's pretty hard not to convince virtually anyone in a hospital of the value of these principles. This suggests that it is, in fact, principles that we need to communicate. The method, a way of achieving goals, becomes secondary.

Wilburn: I would add commitment as an eighth characteristic. Leaders of TQM organizations have to be personally committed to the philosophy and the principles. You also have to be able to transfer that commitment to others in the organization. That speaks to communication, but it also speaks to creating a vision that others want to follow. Commitment is a long-term process. The leader has to recognize that going into TQM and be willing to stick to the commitment.

Prevost: How does the chief executive officer communicate commitment?

Wilburn: By living the philosophy. This communicates to the people you work with on a day-to-day basis, that you are committed to the philosophy and the principles. It involves more than verbal communication. It's communication through actions as well.

Anderson: I'd like to second that. What we're talking about is model-ing behavior. It's paramount that the chief executive officer model the behavior that's expected in a TQM environment.

I'd like to underscore the importance of vision. To me, vision is the overarching concern of leadership—the ability to look down the road to a time when the TQM philosophy has been inculcated throughout the organization. By being able to look into the future, the leader will be able to encourage people during times when things don't go so smoothly. You need to have a good concept of what the hospital is really aiming at and what effects the cultural change will have on the organization. Again, inspiring and establishing a vision is the most important responsibility of leadership of a TQM organization.

Pugh: Trying to inspire a common vision goes beyond communication. We have all seen leaders who embody the seven characteristics, but are out of sync with the organization.

A leader can be restless with the status quo, want change, have high energy, and so on. But until everybody in the organization understands what the hospital is trying to achieve and staff are lined up in the same direction, leadership will not be successful.

Bingham: Jim Prevost said that the leader needs to communicate a vision of what TQM means. I think the leader's responsibilities are even broader. You have to be able to articulate a vision that is relative to the need the hospital is fulfilling in society. Then whether you're meeting with HCFA [Health Care Financing Administration] people or the hospital's medical staff, the leader must keep that vision at the top of the organization's focus. You must integrate TQM concepts through all discussions, at all levels, not just internally but externally with HCFA and others.

Prevost: Well, this concept of vision seems to be a very important characteristic of any hospital leader. Are there special qualities about a leader of a QI hospital? Is it different than being a traditional leader?

Pugh: One hurdle a TQM leader must overcome is the impulse to have all the answers. In many traditional leadership roles, leaders want to have the answer in addition to having the vision. We all know leaders that have all the seven characteristics, but also have all the answers. One difference in a TQM leader is the ability to step back and look to those who are closest to the process or the customer, allowing others to participate in decision-making activities.

Anderson: I think patience is another very significant characteristic. A distinct difference between being a TQM leader as opposed to a traditional leader is that you're not focusing on the bottom line, you're not focusing on quick fixes, you're not focusing on immediate responses. Instead, you're taking a long-term view of the organization, and patience is absolutely essential to accomplish that.

A second difference is that you must believe you can manage without fear. In traditional management, fear is used to drive the organization and to drive subordinates to do what their leaders have in mind. The way you get away from management by

fear is when you become convinced that problems result from dealing with bad processes, not bad people.

Newbold: As a TQM leader I am now more involved in the production function and the details of production as opposed to being more engaged in a number of outside diversification linkages. These outside activities are still important, but I am now focusing more on the details of what is going on inside the hospital. The processes of the hospital have intensified.

I have also become more of a teacher. By this I mean I spend time teaching staff about the fundamental methods of TQM. TQM is a fundamental discipline with a knowledge base. I estimate that I spend something like two hour a day with my senior staff in a continuous learning environment.

Wilburn: I think a TQM leader may develop a better understanding of what goes on internally because there's more participation in processes. While we all had the interest over the years, we probably didn't pay as much attention to internal functions before we actually started using the principles of TQM and looking at customer needs. I don't think we have a stronger internal focus, but we do have a better understanding of what goes on in the hospital.

Bingham: The TQM leader focuses on the internal in a different way than the traditional leader. I'm looking at extended systems more—how what we do inside ties into what we do externally and back to our vision. This linkage is much more clearly in my mind now than it was pre-TQM.

Prevost: This leads us into the issue of the leader's role. How has your role as a chief executive officer changed, say over years one, two, and three of the transition, from what it used to be?

Pugh: I particularly like Deming's quote that says it does little to improve the quality of the house by putting out fires. In the last three years, I've made a tremendous transition away from fire fighting and problem solving in the traditional sense. While there are still problems that need to be solved, I spend far less of my time today than I did four years ago managing crises and much more time in a teaching/learning process with staff members, in planning and talking to traditional customers and internal customers, and in working with departments to understand processes and the TQM principles— that is, transforming the whole organization versus just going out and fixing something that's broken.

Anderson: I agree with Michael. When you look at how organizations have been managed over the years, this emphasis on teaching as the natural responsibility of senior management is quite novel. This is an important distinction that has been established through TQM and is very different from what leaders are used to doing. In my view, "mentoring" is a critical concept for senior administration. The concept of nurturing as a responsibility of executive management is novel and challenging. Frankly, it is a role I enjoy very much.

Prevost: So, what you're saying is that the role of a leader in a QI hospital is changing because there's less fire fighting and less time spent fixing things that are broken and more time spent on QI principles and on mentoring and nurturing others.

Wilburn: There's been more learning going on, and that's a big change. At Bethesda, we've put a major emphasis on the need for senior management and the leaders of the medical staff to learn about TQM, about the various tools that can be used, and about the philosophy and principles. We've put in a lot of time on learning, as well as teaching and coaching, because we had to learn first. That's a major effort in education.

Prevost: In his book *The Fifth Discipline*, Peter Senge talks about the "learning organization." Is that synonymous with a QI organization?

Anderson: It depends on what you're learning. If you were to say that the learning organization is actually a prerequisite to being a TQM organization, that's probably accurate.

Prevost: The rest of you seem to agree with that. When we visited John Bingham's hospital, he talked about being a designer, a steward. Is this similar to Senge's thoughts about leadership in a learning organization?

Bingham: I'm a fan of Senge's ideas on the role of managers or leaders, particularly his idea that the manager must be a designer. Our vision statement "to make Twin Falls the healthiest place in America" is requiring us to look at the design of what's going on in our community, not just in our hospital. So, the leader has a responsibility to set the foundation or vision and make sure it takes into account the extended system.

Our vision has changed my role and how I spend my time. Now, I ask more questions about the extended system—"What's going on in our community?" "How does this impact quality upstream and downstream?" The type of data I look at is also changing because of our vision statement. Our hospital's role is changing to one of designing our community's health care system, being a catalyst in that.

Prevost: Your role has changed, then, inside and outside the hospital. You have become a designer of what occurs in your community's health care system, as well as inside your organization. Do the rest of you agree with John Bingham or do you see it differently?

Newbold: Just a little bit different. It has become very obvious that QI principles are based on prevention. Because the acute care system, as set up in the United States, is based on fixing things that are broken, QI principles don't fit at first with the past experiences of many boards and medical staff leaders. But once they begin designing or visioning a process to improve the health status and quality of life for a defined population, boards and leaders begin to see what might be done in terms of prevention—early detection, screening, going back into the school system, going back to the factors and forces that influence people's lifestyles. From this point of view you begin to see that you can't affect the necessary

changes by yourself and you begin to look at partnering.

Once you have some experience in the QI arena, you begin to shift your thinking about the acute care model we have in the United States. Acquiring some experience in the QI arena oftentimes shifts boards' and leaders' thinking about the organization's mission, purpose, and vision, and where, as Senge says, the biggest leverage points are. When you're talking about quality of life or health status, there's no question about the need to go back to prevention, back to early childhood, or even before birth if you want to get into gene therapy and so on. So QI principles do cause you to fundamentally rethink the future and to challenge, question, and examine the existing acute care system that we've all come to accept over the past thirty years.

Griner: Phil's comment is a good one. I'd like to build on it. There are six acute care hospitals in Rochester, New York. Each of these hospitals has been independently moving along the track of TQM for the last two or three years. In Rochester, we happen to have a history of more cooperation than most communities throughout the country [see page 167 of Chapter 6]. An interesting dynamic is occurring now. All six hospitals have collectively developed a partnership with major industries in Rochester—Xerox, Kodak, and Bausch & Laumb—a partnership that will not only facilitate more rapid movement toward TQM within each of the six institutions but also permit all of us to begin collectively addressing some communitywide issues that we've never looked at as a group.

For example, one concern is Rochester's problem with adolescent pregnancy—20% of women between the ages of 15 and 19 get pregnant every year in Rochester. We have an enormous problem with premature deliveries. Our neonatal intensive care unit is running constantly at a 110% occupancy. Fifty percent of those problems can be prevented through improved prenatal services, both social and medical. We are now coming together as a community of hospitals along with industry and beginning to apply TQM principles to improve these collective communitywide problems.

Newbold: In our neonatal unit, it costs $40,000 to care for premature infants. In many instances, $400, one hundredth of that, in prenatal care would take care of that $40,000 expenditure. Figures like this force you to shift your thinking about prevention.

As we discuss empowerment, visioning, work designing, learning, and so on, it becomes clear that quality is the integrator for many of these concepts. QI is really a catalyst to rethinking the whole acute care system and what we're all about in terms of improving the quality of life for people. In that respect, QI has been an interesting change agent for boards, medical staff leaders, and others. Familarilty with QI principles suddenly forces them to shift their thinking from being driven by reimbursement, money, and so on to considering the system a little differently.

Prevost: Someone's going to have to help me here. Each of your vision statements states that you want to be the best or the premier or the number one in some way or another. At the same time, I'm hearing that you're a spoke in the wheel, a part of a system, and that you need to work with others in that system. I'm having trouble trying to understand this apparent contradiction.

Griner: Competitors in industry share their approaches to TQM. It should be possible to achieve both, Jim. One can be the best. This doesn't mean you have to keep secrets about what you're doing in QI to be the best.

Newbold: The face of competition is changing. When we talked about competition in 1983 or 1984, at the time diagnosis-related groups [DRGs] were introduced, competition meant building as much market share as possible, stepping on your competition's throat if necessary. A hospital's success was measured by market share, filled beds, and more procedures. Seven or eight years have gone by since DRGs were introduced, the medical arms race has escalated, there's been a buildup of pretty good facilities. And yet, after ten years of deregulation, no competitive forces have held down health care costs.

As a result, competition is now being looked at in a different light. The competition that we're focusing on is similar to what Paul Griner and others refer to—that which enables us to develop higher levels of clinical outcomes, attain better levels of service, and arrive at costs that are reasonable, affordable, and competitive. We can achieve these goals not at the expense of our neighbors, but in partnership with our neighbors, to

209

determine exactly how to balance the quality/service/price equation.

Again, the catalyst, the agent that's changed all this, is a sense of competition that is more internally oriented, that enables us to be the best we can possibly be by looking at our work processes and focusing on our clinical outcomes. We have a really different concept of competition than we've had in the past. People are now talking about a more collaborative model of health care. We'll be very competitive in some areas, we'll be regulated in many others, and we'll get along in some others. That's going to be an interesting leadership job.

Wilburn: What I don't understand is whether the TQM focus has been the catalyst that's enabled South Bend or Rochester to move toward more collaboration. I have not seen that occur in Cincinnati.

There are a lot of hospitals talking about TQM, but it has not led to increased servicing of community needs directly out of a TQM framework. More community needs are being addressed because of the problems we are facing as a community. I'm not sure whether in South Bend, for example, collaboration grew out of the TQM movement or if it grew out of the need to address a community problem.

Newbold: I agree that a multitude of factors has influenced the shift to collaboration. At Memorial, we've also been into empowerment for four years and have been doing visioning for the last year or two. But I think that TQM has acted as an integrator between a number of these forces and challenges that we're facing.

Wilburn: The question is not whether these were good things to do, but whether TQM, as we practice it, was the catalyst that led us to look at the community? We're all doing things in the community, but are we doing them because of TQM?

Griner: At least for us in Rochester, the spirit and history of cooperation existed long before the individual hospitals began to apply TQM techniques. But TQM has become a tool for us to more effectively deal with communitywide issues than we have in the past.

Prevost: We seem to be describing a new role for the QI leader, as a systems leader extending beyond the boundaries of the hospital. I think we would all agree that this is a change from the past.

Pugh: QI is also an issue of systems thinking, beginning to understand the interrelatedness of the different systems and optimizing one versus suboptimizing another.

A note of caution. It is easy to use TQM principles to say, "Let's go outside and fix the rest of the world." Our department managers sometimes do this when we talk about the boundaries of the processes they control versus what they want to work on. The majority of early efforts have to be based on what we control, such as improving processes in hospitals because there is such a tremendous opportunity to reduce the cost of waste and rework within those walls. As a competitive strategy at Parkview, we have dramatically cut our marketing budget and external promotion so we can begin focusing internally. We are attracting physicians and customers by the quality of what we do. This does not mean I do not worry about the outside, the outputs of our hospital, or what comes in, or about trying to improve the existing health care system. But our major emphasis has to be inside the boundaries of what we control.

Bingham: While I agree that hospitals have to focus internally on the processes we can control, I don't believe this focus is enough—even if what we do internally is done very, very well. We won't significantly impact the health status of people until we start to look externally as well. And so, I maintain that the hospital has a role to be a catalyst, to ensure that TQM is extended out into the community and to other providers, including the competition, in order to improve people's health status. It is not enough to use TQM as a competitive advantage; that doesn't achieve what hospitals are in business for—improving people's health.

Pugh: Well said. I don't disagree. But in talking about the role of hospital leaders, I don't think you should use the principles of TQM as an excuse to go out externally from the organization. It's an alluring sort of role— becoming involved in the bigger system. But a lot of our time needs to be spent internally. When you work on processes inside, it will lead you outside. But, to go out and use TQM as a springboard to change the health care world before we change ourselves probably won't work any better than all the other springboards tried before.

IMPLEMENTING QI—THE ROLLOUT

Prevost: While there might not be a single best strategy for implementing QI, is there a general sequence of transitional steps for successfully rolling out QI in hospitals?

Pugh: First, I'd like to clarify how each of us operationally defines TQM in terms of rolling it out.

Prevost: Fair enough, why don't you begin, Michael, by giving us your definition.

Pugh: Well, two weeks ago I heard Ed Baker at Ford say that he wished the word "quality" had never been associated with what Ford's doing. What they're really talking about at Ford is a fundamental change in management theory and organizational theory based on what Dr Deming has been teaching and thinking about for a number of years. Unfortunately, so much of what's out there under the guise of TQM is the same old stuff just repackaged under the term CQI. I think how TQM is rolled out is going to reflect the model each of us works with.

Prevost: How do the rest of you feel about this?

Newbold: I disagree. A new management model doesn't necessarily have an end point. It's not focused on doing something. We've had dozens of new management models: management by walking around, theory x/theory y, and management by objectives. These are all management theories, but they aren't focused on an end product. TQM is focused on better clinical outcomes and meeting customer requirements, which is different from just putting a new management theory in place.

Newbold: I suspect that Ford is doing what it's doing to improve quality. Whether or not you call it a new management theory, I think it's the means toward the end. The end is being more competitive because of quality.

Anderson: Wright-Patterson's approach and our definition of quality is, in fact, meeting or exceeding customer expectations. Obviously, being process-driven, being customer-focused, encouraging teamwork, and using statistical process control are included under this definition as well. All these things are part and parcel of our definition of quality. But the major point is that quality is not some extrinsic activity as we traditionally define it.

Bingham: Essentially, we're using Deming's 14 points, that's Magic Valley's focus.

Wilburn: Well, at Bethesda, we've been using Deming plus the newer innovations that the Japanese have put into TQM. We're trying to utilize all the tools that we can to improve our services in addition to focusing on customer expectations and processes.

Pugh: Well, I didn't give you Parkview's full definition. It's continuously improving services that meet or exceed the expectations of customers.

Anderson: That definition is totally consistant with ours.

Prevost: Can a hospital expect to achieve the transition with the use of QI methods and problem-solving tools, or must its goal be a completely transformed management system?

Newbold: When I speak at hospital seminars and retreats, one of the first things I always ask is, "What are you trying to do with this whole movement? Are you just trying to get a little bit better, or are you interested in fundamentally changing your organization over a period of three to six years?" I get a 50/50 response to that question. A lot of participants think about the question and say, "We think we're good now, we just want to get a little better." Others say, "We would like to be a very different organization in 1995 or 2000 from what we are today." They each list the characteristics of the kind of organization they want to be, and they all have their own approach to it.

I suspect that how you answer that question will have a lot to do with how you roll out your TQM plan, how much intensity is generated, and a whole lot of other factors. At Memorial, we selected the transformation model. Basically we're trying to achieve a new organization.

Prevost: Should those interested in achieving CQI seek the transformation model or will focusing on the methods and tools of QI be sufficien to bring about the change?

Anderson: Executive managemen can employ some of the methods o TQM, and its initial goal may just b to better the organization by doin these things. All that is accomplishec

I think, is a delay in the cultural transformation. This transformation will occur anyway and senior management will become committed because, once they get involved in TQM, it will take them over simply because TQM works. The synthesis of statistical process control, teamwork, and process-driven activities is inevitably going to change the organization.

Pugh: This issue is like the "project" versus the "philosophy" question. "Is QI just another project that senior management delegates or is this a philosophy of organizational management, a management theory?" We're seeing the project option played out in a number of hospitals. I don't know if it's effective, but I do think it often exists. But if it's a management theory based on philosophical principles, it becomes part of the organization and how you do business and you'll get a tranformed hospital.

Prevost: None of the six hospitals represented here reflects the project option. Each of you seems to be moving toward the total transformation of your organization.

Bingham: I'm not sure it's an option in the long run. A project hospital will not be able to compete with those hospitals that successfully achieve a total transformation.

Panzer: The end result may be spotty in an organization that's only partially implementing TQM. You might have wonderful quality within department lines, but miserable quality in terms of coordination.

For example, the leader of our emergency department was recruited about two years ago and embodied virtually all seven characteristics we spoke about earlier. He made tremendous changes in quality within the emergency department that look a lot like the output of a QI team. But the coordination of the emergency room and other areas in the hospital is less well developed because those areas are not ready to talk about quality and because the joint efforts aren't in place.

So, you can achieve the two- or three-year milestones of TQM with alternate methods, but you'll find barriers to its growth. Transformation has to begin in an integrated fashion.

Prevost: How does hospital leadership decide that the time is right to make this journey?

Wilburn: We sent a number of our people to Deming's four-day seminar, and we had a lot of discussions about TQM philosophy and principles following the seminar. We reached a consensus among our leadership that TQM was something we ought to pursue.

Panzer: Top-level commitment has to come first. You have to see it at the chief executive officer level. I haven't seen boards not be supportive of leadership's commitment. Education is second. TQM is a discipline, there is a specific, known methodology. You must spend the time to learn it. It can take hundreds of hours for an organization to really learn, and you never stop learning. You're learning something all the time. So I think Tom Wilburn's approach about education and building that top-level commitment and support is correct. Top management need to be educated in TQM methodology and discipline before they really work with an organization and take the steps necessary to fully transform the organization. The right time to roll out TQM is when the chief executive officer is committed and education has been achieved to a certain extent.

Anderson: TQM is a top-down-driven activity, but there's a very key point here. TQM gets away from the concept that the chief executive officer is the one to decide everything. Senior management has to be as highly conversant, knowledgeable, and dedicated to TQM as the chief executive officer. You've got to get TQM anchored at that level before you can really cascade it through the rest of the organization. At Wright Patterson, senior management forms our Quality Council, which used to be our Executive Committee. I think the anchoring process in senior management, which is really an involved process, is critical to the success of the transformation process.

Griner: About five years before we began to talk about TQM at our hospital, we wanted the medical staff to recognize that our quality assurance (QA) program did not exist because it was required by the Joint Commission or by the New York Department of Health. Instead we wanted the medical staff to recognize that, in terms of care and responsibility, our QA program represented us as professionals. Until we, as a medical staff, became comfortable with that concept, we wouldn't have gotten anywhere with the more formal, systematic approaches that we're now taking with TQM.

Prevost: Would you say that there has

to be an effective working relationship between the administration and the medical staff before initiating QI?

Griner: You need to have trust between the medical staff and the administration.

Newbold: When I talk to people about implementing TQM in their organization, I try to give them some notion of what they're getting themselves into. It's hard to do—implementing TQM is so experiential in nature. But as a rule of thumb, I always say that initially senior management needs to spend about two hours a day educating themselves. If they're really not interested in operations and making operational changes, they would be well advised not to pursue implementing TQM, because it's harder to jump start these TQM efforts after you've tried it and failed. You really have to think this whole process through pretty carefully, and if there are some trust issues between the medical staff and administration, these should be dealt with first.

Another distressing issue is the turnover of chief executive officers in the field. I don't know how a hospital can introduce TQM with any degree of continuity if you're changing administrators or senior leadership every two or three years.

Again, I tell people that three to six years really means three to six years, not three to six months. Raising expectations to an inappropriate level is about as big a problem as I see among people involved in implementing TQM. In the health care field, we don't have any experience of doing something for three to six years, except maybe budgeting. We just don't stick with things for long periods of times. So when you say TQM is different, that it will take three to six years, you get a lot of skeptical reactions. I encourage people to have a realistic picture of the time commitments, the change in thinking, the new approaches, the new management philosophy, and their new role. They're better off waiting until they accept this realistic picture before they begin to implement TQM.

Pugh: I don't know where you get the six years—it's more like three years to a lifetime.

Newbold: I spent a day in a meeting with Dr Juran and I asked him that question. He had a lot of reasons why six years was realistic. He believes that you should start seeing some successes from your efforts at three years. He had a whole lot of reasons, too, why results wouldn't happen before three years.

Bingham: I'd like to expand a bit on Phil Newbold's comments about the need for CEO stability. It's more than the CEO. There also has to be senior management and board stability. You need to address important issues such as whether you're going to have turnover in any key positions or whether new board members are coming on. You might want to stabilize your board and senior management team before you begin to implement TQM. Also, if the hospital is in financial distress, or you have to deal with financial issues that require some very tough decisions, it would be very, very difficult to embark on implementing TQM.

Wilburn: Most of us look for a quick fix; it's really common. People still see TQM as something that, if you do it right, can be done very quickly. It just isn't so. I think that's something we need to emphasize for those that embark on the journey. Implementing TQM is going to take a while. That point has to be clear.

Prevost: At the time of our site visits, most of you, in retrospect, thought the QI training provided to staff covered too many things in the beginning. Most of you felt that it might have been better to focus at first on QI principles, with more in-depth training on the use of methods and problem-solving tools occurring later in a "just-in-time" fashion.

Many of you said you should have planned more at the outset, that planning needed to take place side by side with training. You all had stories about how some of your early teams got training, but didn't quite know where to go with it, while other teams seemed to know where they were going, but didn't have the training. Do several important things in this transitional sequence need to be coupled, such as training and planning?

Wilburn: After we decided to commit, said we were going to do this, we formed pilot teams that were diagnostic in nature. We wanted to determine what barriers and opportunities existed in our organization to TQM and what would keep TQM from moving through the organization so that top management could facilitate that movement. In some instances, we overtrained team members. By the time they got to use the tools they'd learned, they'd forgotten what the tools meant. As part of our roll out, we made adjustments to the team education activities.

Panzer: We started with the project team model at Strong, but abandoned it fairly quickly after we entered a lull. We restarted our efforts with more heavy-duty planning and cascade training. Eventually, much further down the road, we got back to project teams. I think the same sequence is repeated in other organizations.

Newbold: We did exactly the same thing at Memorial. It's interesting that you had that same experience we had. We call it, "We've got a thousand people dressed up for the dance, but no dance to go to." Staff were all trained and ready to go, and there just weren't enough project teams for all these folks to serve on. So, we moved quickly into quality planning.

Pugh: Looking back, one of the things we wish we'd done differently, or done sooner, was to spend more time in the planning stage.

Since all six of us started about the same time, in 1987 or 1988, most of us began operating under what I call the "critical mass theory," which says if we educate everybody about QI the result will be like nuclear fusion: critical mass will come together and the organization will be transformed. It's the same thing as dressing everybody up for the dance with no dance to take them to.

In retrospect, one of the big turning points for us was moving away from the "critical mass theory" and deciding what was important for the organization to work on—improving the five key systems that run organizationwide. But none of us knew at first the importance of marshalling our resources, giving everybody an organizational focus. A lot of our confusion was a sign of the times.

Another big trap that we fell into at Parkview was to create a lot of fanfare about TQM being the new way of doing things. This raised staff's expectations that a big, positive change was on the horizon. But this also puts a tremendous amount of pressure on the department managers. They were caught in the middle. Many developed the attitude of "this too shall pass." We made a major faux pas in the beginning by not bringing in the middle manager, a really key person, to help us lead.

Newbold: It's pretty obvious what builds commitment and what doesn't. Education alone doesn't build commitment. You've got to practice, practice, practice—put the training in place and practice a dozen times over in order to realize any benefit.

Anderson: The military is designed for action. Therefore, when we got into TQM, we intended to solve the problems right away. That was the approach that we had envisioned. It became obvious after a short time that this attitude was absolutely incongrous with the whole concept of TQM.

Second, we began to recognize that it's essential that one have training before trying to form process action teams. At a minimum, the leader of the team has got to be trained for the team to operate effectively. Many of our first teams were given a problem to solve without the proper education and skills. The bad thing that came out of all this, o course, was discouragement.

The question that hospital staff will be asking is: "Is TQM really a fundamental change that you're preaching, or is it just another 'flavor of the month?'" If staff see somewhat shaky outcomes after you initiate changes, then they get the sense that they've gotten another flavor of the month—and they've had too many of those. We must ensure that staff recognize that TQM is not a quick-fix method and that this represents a fundamental alteration in how we do business, not just a management fad.

Prevost: Should implementation of the transition come from the existing organizational structure or should changes occur in that structure in order to support this change process?

Newbold: I see no reason for an organization to change its organizational structure.

Bingham: I agree, with one exception. One of the lessons we learned was the importance of a full-time coach. We should have brought a full-time coach on from the moment we started, but we assumed that our QA person or a senior management team member could serve in that role—it wasn't enough.

Wilburn: There has to be coordination. This doesn't necessitate changing the organization's structure, but it does necessitate greater communication and coordination between managers and leaders in the organization so they understand what's going on and why their people are participating.

Panzer: At Strong, we are rolling out TQM in the structure we had in place.

We have decentralized management of clinical services and centralized clinical supports, such as data analysis and QA. Our roll out to the clinical environment involves the clinical chief, nursing clinical chief, and the program administrator together. So we train them jointly in that structure. I imagine if we didn't have a decentralized structure, we would have done it within whatever structure existed.

Anderson: When you're dealing with quality, you have to make it a part of the overall organization. Most importantly, you have to involve those people who run the organization already, inculcate in them your organization's particular philosophy. This way you don't have to come up with another parallel structure to evaluate, rather you utilize more effectively the organizational structure that you have already.

Prevost: Are there any other issues related to the roll out of TQM that you would like to discuss?

Newbold: I'm just wondering if the rest of you are having the same problems using patient satisfaction surveys as a measurement or key quality indicator. There are so many work processes and so many different factors that affect patient satisfaction. Staff work and work and they try and try but these scores don't seem to improve. Staff don't feel close enough to the patients sometimes to make a real difference in patient satisfaction scores. At Memorial, we're struggling with this issue all the time.

A related issue is how much to survey. I've had 16 requests for new patient satisfaction surveys, and five or six surveys are going out to patients already. Patients are calling to tell me they are being surveyed to death.

Bingham: I don't think patient satisfaction surveys are anywhere near as valuable as I once thought they were for a number of reasons. One, I think there are a lot of biases statistically that make the data incorrect. Second, the surveys do not provide real-time data. Finally, our systems are fraught with process improvement problems that hospital staff are already aware of. We don't really need to go to the customer to tell us where improvements need to be made. It doesn't take a genius to know that a half-hour wait time for a chest x-ray is not going to please the customer. I think our hospital needs to devote money and energy into improving the processes that we already know need our attention.

Wilburn: We're taking a different tack. To understand what our customers expect, we believe we have to survey them. But we decided that we're not as good as we ought to be at asking the correct questions of patients, so we've employed professionals to do it. We hired Gallup and they are attaining patient feedback through phone interviews.

Anderson: One of the most difficult things to do in this whole business is find out what your customer wants. Although it is essential to find out what the patient or other customer wants, it's difficult because the users, or patients, do not articulate their expectations.

Let me give you an example of something we did at Wright-Patterson very early in our TQM roll out. We knew we needed to find out what the customers want, but how could we do it? There's only one thing to do—ask them. Well, how do you go about asking them? We decided to survey our customers and find out "what is the most important thing that we, as a medical center, can do for you." We devised a survey for inpatients and distributed it outside the base commissary and base exchange. We wanted feedback from those who didn't use our facilities as well as those who did. Then, we gave a similar survey to hospital staff and asked "what is the most important thing that patients want from us."

When we compared the answers, staff responses were very different from those of patients. Staff responses were "give patients good medical care" and "utilize the very finest medical equipment possible to cure diseases." But patients' responses were "we can't get people to answer telephones" and "we can't get appointments." Seventy-five percent of the patients said that all they wanted was to get into our health care system. They said they were sure our staff would take good care of them once they got into the medical center, but there was no access.

Pugh: I fall in the middle of the argument concerning patient satisfaction surveys. You cannot find out what patients really want just through a patient survey. You have got to use other tactics as well, such as focus group interviews. Simple surveys are great for spotting special causes or obvious areas for improvement, but I am not sure they are very good for long-term improvement.

Bingham: We're changing our customer research to be more future oriented. We're getting away from asking "What process did you not like when you were in the hospital two months ago?" Instead, we are asking patients to describe, for example, "the ideal x-ray experience." We are trying to get out ahead of the patient as opposed to looking back historically.

BARRIERS/RESISTANCE

Prevost: What are the major internal barriers or resistances to the transition and how have you successfully resolved them?

Newbold: A fundamental shift has occurred in my thinking about quality, about my whole management style. It's a shift away from blaming people and toward looking at work processes as the reason, the root cause, for quality problems or for operations not going well. I've had all the textbook learning, the MBA programs about theory x and theory y, but I still catch myself asking "Who's responsible?" when something doesn't go right. We in health care keep going back to that same knee-jerk reaction time and time again.

Now hospitals are beginning to ask why, not who, and to focus on work processes as the root cause of problems rather than people. As Deming says, driving out fear and blame is at the absolute heart of TQM. When people ask, "Who's accountable?" what they really mean is "Who's to blame?" Once our thinking shifts, we'll start asking different questions like "Why do we seem to have the kinds of outcomes or problems that we're having?" rather than "Who's

responsible?" Focusing on work processes rather than people is our biggest, most fundamental barrier, one we're still trying to get up and over. We confront it just about every day we manage.

Anderson: Because we're in an authoritarian culture—by definition, the military is an authoritarian culture—it was very difficult for our staff to adopt an innovative approach like TQM, especially for people who have not experienced it at all.

It is the fear of losing control, authority that is the most threatening. This fear of losing control is probably worse at the middle management level than any place else, which is probably true in any organization. It is difficult because those managers are used to saying "do it," and no questions are asked. Now TQM says the employee is important and not only has the right but a responsibility to ask, "Is this a nonvalue-added activity that we're embarking upon? What can we do to improve it?"

Wilburn: I agree with John. Middle managers are most resistant to the fear of losing control. In many instances, middle managers are people who have just come into a position of power, so to speak, and they're reluctant to share that power with their staff. We've found that employees understand this pretty quickly. We're sure middle managers understand it, too. But there's resistance to it because it does result in diminution of control.

Another barrier we've encountered is TQM being seen as an add-on activity and an extra time commitment. Many people see the tools themselves as barriers. Even though they were educated about the tools, training alone does not leave them truly proficient in their use. When you have a quick-fix attitude and want to get something done, the tools become barriers because it takes time to learn them.

Bingham: I agree that fear, time, and, as I mentioned earlier, the lack of a coach are all barriers to implementing TQM. I'd like to add the lack of a well-articulated rollout plan to that list. Magic Valley used a generic plan without sufficiently customizing it to what we were doing. Having not thought through the process very well caused some confusion. Staff are not certain what the next steps are. This has been a big barrier at Magic Valley.

Another barrier I'd like to stress is the failure of senior management to be stewards to department managers and midlevel people. Because we did not coach and mentor and were not stewards to our middle management through this process, we have hit, as many of you have also experienced, middle management resistance. If I could do it again, I would spend much more time being a steward to these people, helping them understand what TQM is about, and reassuring them that their job is not going to be eliminated, although it will be much different.

Prevost: What do you say to middle management when they bring these concerns to you?

Bingham: Well, the first thing to do is to build trust and create an atmosphere in which they'll bring their concerns to you. There was a lot go-ing on during our TQM roll out that I didn't hear about and should have heard about. So, the first thing to do is make sure the culture allows people to come and tell you what they're really thinking about, to admit they don't want to lose control, or that they sense they're going to be out of a job. The second thing is time. Senior managment has to spend more time with middle managers listening to their concerns.

Pugh: One of the big barriers, I think, is our inability to articulate to middle management what this transformed state will look like and what their jobs in that state will be. The clue is to give them an idea of what they're going to be doing on a day-to-day basis, to translate that vision down to the practical. We've wrestled a lot with changing the structure of how we report, what we reward, and what types of behaviors we encourage. For example, we make an effort to let everybody in the organization know that team participation, working at processes, and talking to customers—other departments—are the types of behaviors that we want to see more of.

I ask my staff a rhetorical question at QI education sessions: "What would the job of an RN be like in a hospital where all the systems were designed right and worked right the first time?" Nobody knows the answer. Nobody's ever seen it. How does a hospital totally committed to the principles of QI function? We all know that the principles of QI need to function on a daily basis, but what do those principles look like acted out and how do they work? How is a QI hospital organized? Nobody knows, no one has seen one yet.

After three years, our six hospitals are probably about 10%-15% along in the transition. There's a lot still unknown and unknowable. This creates fear in the organization—in part, for middle managers. A lot of the leader's job is to try to drive that fear out, by modeling behaviors, admitting mistakes, coaching. Coaching and stewarding our managers, that encouraging function that John Bingham talks about, is an important activity. It's a key part in overcoming some barriers. Spend time with middle managers, let them know it's okay to make mistakes, it's okay to have doubts.

Newbold: We do a couple exercises during our awareness training. First, we ask all staff to think a little bit, envision, what a Memorial would be like if it had very quality, for example, in the year 2000. Staff then draw a picture of this vision—you can't use words, you have to draw pictures. People come up with just incredible pictures about what the future Memorial looks like. This exercise makes them think about a brighter future that is free of defects, where quality is very high, and staff are fully empowered and practicing their profession at the highest level.

We do another exercise for managers. A group of managers are asked to identify the top ten quality problems in the hospital. Then we ask those managers that have been around for ten years what the top ten quality problems were ten years ago. We might pull out meeting minutes from previous years to find other

kinds of issues. Generally, seven or eight out of the ten current problems are the same problems we had ten years ago. Usually they're not big problems, but it's those little stones in your shoe that drive you crazy day after day after day.

This exercise makes managers begin to ask "How can we continue to expect things to get better when we're doing things the same way every year?" Doing the same thing over and over again but expecting different results is one of the definitions of insanity. At this point, we ask staff: "In ten years do you want the exact same ten problems that you're wrestling with or might we look at a different approach to problem-solving and clinical outcomes?" We give them some stories about what things might be like if we take a different approach. This kind of experiential learning is often useful because we can't do a very good job of actively painting the future.

Pugh: The "one-shot approach" to training and education can be another barrier. Often we'll teach staff something once and expect them to pick up on it. A lot of education, as Tom Wilburn mentioned, needs to be continuous. This includes the formal education of department managers and others who are going to be leaders in the organization. Although self-study needs to be part of this continuous learning, self-study by itself will not necessarily work. Adults learn in different ways. Not everybody sits down and reads a book. Some prefer a video, some learn by doing. You need to build an education program that allows for these different learning styles and that hits the key principles time and time and time again. Learning won't happen in one shot.

This next barrier is a little more esoteric and has to do with the way hospitals are organized. The traditional hospital structure, departmentalization by professional group, is a major barrier to QI because of the pull between loyalty to profession and loyalty to the larger organization. You end up trying to optimize your department against other departments.

At Parkview, we did a couple simple things to address this issue. For example, about 18 months ago we took all the ancillary, support, and nursing departments and put them in two divisions. We no longer have a traditional division of nursing. We now have two vice-presidents of patient services—both happen to be RNs. Getting people in a common division to sit down together with the same leader has made a tremendous difference in our ability to break down traditional barriers. We don't have the issue of nursing against the rest of the world that you see in most hospital organizations.

Prevost: Are there any other barriers that haven't been mentioned?

Panzer: The lack of science behind health care TQM is a major barrier. There is no evidence of what works when and whether the concept as a whole works. We have a lot of scientists at Strong. They all ask "How do we know this is going to work in our institution?" And their universal response to the answers we give them is "That's pretty lousy evidence you've got there." The fact that widgets are being made better at Xerox doesn't convince them. That's one of the reasons, we think, that so few organizations are very far along in the transformation—particularly teaching hospitals.

Prevost: Is your leadership making a commitment to QI despite what they feel is lack of solid evidence of its success in health care?

Panzer: Commitment is being made with what some would call risk, yes.

Anderson: One of the barriers we're facing is caused by a perception of TQM as a philosophy that breeds zealots, rather than as a scientific approach to management. In some instances, people are really turned off by the zeal with which most of us involved in TQM promote it.

Prevost: Sounds like forget the science, make a leap of faith and full speed ahead!

Anderson: One of our concerns is how to show that TQM makes good sense. It's not a set of principles you come to believe in because Deming prescribed it, but because it makes good sense and it works. We've found that staff really don't understand what we're talking about, including some people at high levels.

We're trying two models to help us through some of these barriers. One is departmental task analysis in which we analyze what we're doing in terms of customers. (See page 53 of Chapter 2.) This approach helps departments understand the importance of asking their customers what they want. Departments use this customer knowledge to come up with a vision and mission for their particular area of the organization. Departments begin to look at themselves more critically using these particular tools. We've found this to be a very effective mechanism for getting staff to buy in to TQM.

Pugh: Another barrier is the idea that medicine is special and has a higher ethic so none of these concepts apply. In reality, most of what happens at Parkview on a day-to-day basis is not any different than what happens in other organizations that deal with supplies and paper and scheduling and moving things around.

At the same time, the clinician-patient relationship, around which everything in a hospital is geared, is special. It's based on professional knowledge and experience. The time a clinician works with a patient is a magic moment—a special, special moment. But that moment takes place in a flash of white each day. The rest of the time, things go on. Getting our organization to understand that we can learn from outside health care was a big barrier, initially. You can learn a lot from the outside—ways of moving inventory, ways of scheduling, ways of organizing patient care functions. It's not as big a leap of faith, I think, as we like to make it out to be.

Panzer: I think one of the ways of overcoming the barrier of disbelief is logic. Because our systems are more complex and in more disarray than those in industry, there's good reason to think that this approach is going to be more effective in health care.

Prevost: What seems to emerge at some point, typically two or three years into the transition, is a lull or a

stagnant period. That's puzzling. I believe that has occurred at each of your hospitals.

Why does this lull or stagnant period happen? How should people in other hospitals across the country understand it, especially if they're inexperienced in QI?

Pugh: Implementing TQM is hard. It's hard work, it's hard to do. You don't get the instant rewards that we all hope we'll get. At some point in time, some questions get raised about whether TQM is worthwhile or not.

Prevost: Is this lull something one would expect to follow from the initial enthusiasm?

Bingham: Initially, TQM makes so much sense. When someone presents the principles to you at a Deming seminar, or another similar program, you think "we can do this in 18 months."

So everyone charges out, and you're on this high plain. Everything's going well, it feels good, and people are talking differently to each other. But then, all of a sudden, everyone starts realizing how hard TQM is—that it's not simple. All of Deming's 14 points are very difficult to implement. This is when people start stalling, they do a dive. And you spend a while there, in a free-fall. At this point, some people check out. They say, "I'm not willing to do that. This is too hard. I won't learn that much."

Wilburn: Our experience has been that people, particularly the doubters in your senior management group, will begin to ask about the return. It's the old thinking—"How much are we investing? What are we getting back?"

Pugh: Is it a cost issue?

Wilburn: Yes. One committee member asked, "We've invested $800,000 on this, what the hell have we gotten out of it?" Cost becomes the question. I asked the rest of the steering committee if they wanted to "buy out" of TQM. I said that if we wanted to call a halt to the process, this was the time to do it. But except for the individual who raised the issue, we got unanimous agreement to continue.

Anderson: As I mentioned before, some organizations are bottom-line oriented. If you get into TQM and you don't do something about that bottom-line perspective quickly, one of two things happen. Some people will say, "Let's get out of this, it's obviously not an effective approach." Or this perspective could drive you to do things you wouldn't usually do. For instance, it drove us at Wright-Patterson to the concept of "fast PATs," or doing things rapidly such as using a tool without appropriate training. When this kind of approach is taken and the desired improvements don't materialize, discouragement occurs. People get discouraged and TQM efforts begin to fall apart.

Prevost: Are there other ways to deal with this lull in the transition?

Pugh: Go outside and visit another hospital that's suffered through the same thing. Talk to those people, see how they dealt with it or get some additional education. Bring in a consultant. I'd do something to stimulate and reeducate senior leadership.

Anderson: One of the things that helps, especially initially, is to work on some smaller processes where victories can be readily achieved. If you get some victories, then you're able to encourage and stimulate people to stay in for the long run.

Pugh: Maybe the way that we went about it created some of the lull. Most of us went for unfocused, mass education. Maybe those who follow us won't experience some of that lull if they have a more clear idea of how to roll out TQM.

MEDICAL STAFF INVOLVEMENT

Prevost: When we conducted our on-site visits to the six hospitals, there seemed to be a lack of medical staff involvement. That's a possible overstatement, but it raises a question. When is the best time to fully engage physicians in the transition?

Bingham: We decided not to involve physicians early on. That was the advice we received from a physician consultant, Dr Paul Batalden. So we didn't involve physicians, with the exception of a few that really expressed an interest and were very motivated to learn about TQM. Yet Dr Paul Miles, a pediatrician on our hospital board, said he would have involved physicians from the start if Magic Valley could do it again.

Prevost: You might feel differently now for the reasons you just mentioned, but I gather there were some good reasons why you essentially waited to engage physicians.

Newbold: It's hard enough to launch TQM to 2,000 employees much less tackle the medical staff at the same time. I was more interested in removing resistance to TQM than in building support. I felt that if we could show physicians that TQM is based on scientific principles, that it follows a logical problem-solving sequence, and that hospital staff were united in their focus on quality and patient care outcomes, they would get behind it very strongly.

Very early on, our concern was to make sure the medical staff had a basic understanding or awareness of TQM. It is pretty difficult to launch into an hour on Deming's 14 points. Everybody starts looking at their watches, and they can't wait to get out. So, instead we went through this long process of giving physicians five-to ten-minute little bites about the quality efforts underway at Memorial and the principles behind it. They heard about TQM gradually over time.

Sometime after this, an ER problem was brought up at a medical staff committee meeting. The same old problem-solving appoach kicked in: "Who's responsible? Let's blame somebody." It was suggested that we wait on that approach, and I began to describe another method that involved looking at work processes, setting customer requirements, developing and measuring with quality indicators, and using quality tools. Afterward, everyone said that the approach I described was the best thing that had happened at that meeting in the last five years they had with the committee.

Physicians are hungry for something besides the same old approaches to the same old problems. But it took a lot of groundwork before I could mention customer require-

ments at that meeting, before physicians would recognize what I was talking about. By dropping bits of information to them over time, physicians were eventually able to say to themselves, "Oh yeah, I've heard about customer requirements before. Work processes? Yeah, I've heard that all work is a process and that we might examine how processes fit together." This recognition took as long as it did because physicians are not employees. They come in and out of the hospital at various times, and you just have to make the most of the time you have with them.

Anderson: We have a unique situation at Wright-Patterson because we are in a closed-panel group practice. This has made a lot of difference because the physicians are part and parcel of the hospital organization.

But I've been giving a lot of thought to how you could approach physicians who essentially use the hospital as a workplace. It's essential that we find ways of approaching TQM that are of interest to them. They're concerned about their offices. Why not train their office people in TQM so that physicians can see a definitive kind of improvement? We have a golden opportunity to seduce them in this manner. Once you can do that, then you'll have them in the fold. Physicians are not going to concern themselves, necessarily, with the hospital and its problems unless they directly affect them.

Wilburn: We wanted the medical staff involved in TQM from the beginning. One of the things we did at Bethesda was provide support to physicians in their offices, the very thing you suggest, John. Other methods we used included having three members of the medical staff serve on our Quality 1 Steering Committee from the beginning. (Quality 1 is the name we use for our TQM effort.) We also held a medical staff retreat to inform the department and section heads of what we were doing; people from Harvard Community Health Plan came to talk to them about TQM. We asked for volunteers and got 23 from the medical staff to work on clinical applications of TQM.

An initial impulse, when moving what might be called a "production system" into a health care setting, is to stay away from clinical processes. I ran into that back in the 1960s when I was brought in to apply industrial management techniques to health care. At the time, my boss wanted to apply these techniques in the laboratory, tray assembly line, dietary, and environmental services but stay away from the doctors. But if you look at why hospitals are in business, it is to provide medical care. And staying away from the doctors or the medical staff doesn't make sense if you're looking to improve what you do.

We've had clinical project teams going now for over two years with good results. For example, a team involving emergency physicians, pulmonologists, and internists has affected the treatment of asthma patients in the emergency department. Another team has conducted an excellent review of the administration of prophylactic antibiotics. Right now we have seven clinical issues being addressed by the medical staff. One is cesarean sections, another is hip replacements. A third is fertility, or rather the process in place at the infertility clinic. That team started out trying to determine how they could reduce the cost in the clinic. It's difficult to price services. In examining that process, the team figured out that we had an eight-week backlog of customers we were turning off. Now the emphasis has changed from trying to reduce the cost of the clinic to trying to ensure a more effective process. That's the real answer anyway.

Anderson: Do you have nonphysicians on these teams?

Wilburn: We have nonphysicians and physicians. One thing we're addressing is how to minimize and make useful the amount of time physicians spend on teams. Because when you talk about attending physicians working on teams, you're talking about dollars out of their pocket. So, you have to use their time effectively. That's been a major challenge. But, to be honest, I think the best results are going to come from clinical teams.

Pugh: The issue of involving the medical staff will differ with every hospital that goes through this process. What's important in the decision is how the medical staff interfaces with the board and management, what the organization's key problems are, why the hospital is embarking on TQM, and so on. So you're going to see more than one model for involving the medical staff.

We decided up-front not to involve medical staff members at first other than as suppliers and customers to different processes that are important to them. We wanted to work on things that were important to them.

We have a relationship with the medical staff that is pretty typical in a community hospital. A hospital is the place where they work, and the amount of time they choose to spend in other activities such as TQM is dependent upon how much it will enhance their practice, their loyalty to the hospital, and if it captures their imagination.

Because hospitals are built on systems that allow the practice of medicine to take place, I strongly believe that unless you fix the underlying systems, the clinician/patient interface does not work, or it works despite the way your systems work. We wanted to make sure we could make improvements in those underlying systems and show improvements to our physicians and others as evidence that TQM works. I wanted to make sure we had a foundation to build on and proof that TQM worked before setting out to change what physicians do. We did not want to risk that physicians would dismiss TQM as another QA requirement imposed by the Joint Commission.

I agree that the greatest improvements in the long term will be in the clinical area as we determine what are the best current methods of clinical management. That is ultimately where we need to go because a tremendous amount of variation exists. It is not the fault of physicians. We have never given them good feedback on how or what they were doing.

Prevost: Strong has a program titled "Innovations in Patient Care" (IPC). I think it supports what we've observed—that nothing intrinsic about TQM conflicts with the way physicians

think or practice. In fact, there's a lot in common. A very interesting change occurred at Strong with their IPC program. Bob, why don't you give us an overview.

Panzer: The IPC program started in 1986 at a budget and planning committee meeting. The committee was trying to build a reward linkage with the medical school faculty who worked in the hospital. They wanted a reward system that was compatible with our culture. They came up with a program that allowed academic people to lead a study of potential new clinical practice and, thereby, help figure out how to improve our services. So the hospital put up $150,000 per year.

A letter went out from the chief executive officer to every physician, nurse, and administrator on staff, residents and fellows, inviting them to send in ideas for projects for between $5,000 and $15,000. We reviewed the proposals and funded those that met our goals, including an impact on cost and quality.

What was surprising was the number of high-quality responses and who responded. Most first-year responses came from academic generalists, pediatricians, and internists. But at least half the responses that year, and in most subsequent years, have come from department leaders proposing a project that would improve a service. Basically, the IPC has become a way to get physicians directing QI teams, to have research investigations redesigning parts of the hospital system.

The surprise has been the extent to which the IPC program is compatible with the medical school culture. It has gotten the medical school bought into the themes of TQM—accepting change, accepting innovation, not tolerating the status quo—and become the new approach for resolving disagreements. When staff come in and say, "I believe my way is the better way to do this . . ." management can now reply, "It's a close call, why don't you answer the question with a pilot."

Prevost: Sounds like the IPC program made a bridge between the Shewhart cycle and health services research.

Panzer: Yes, and it is, like many of our efforts, a decentralized program in which each of the proposers becomes a leader of the project. The IPC looks like it will be a core piece of the way we'll do CQI in the future. It's one of the more effective ways we can make improvements in the clinical setting.

Anderson: In organized medicine, we're using practice parameters more and more—an accursed concept to most physicians, absolutely accursed. Nevertheless, most physicians recognize practice parameters as a reality. This is a golden opportunity for those of us in TQM to make a significant, palliative impact because what we're talking about is decreasing variation. That's what practice parameters are all about, and that's certainly something we in TQM have some expertise in.

Wright-Patterson, like Bethesda, involved the medical staff early in our TQM efforts. It's been our experience that the earlier you get the clinical staff involved, the better it is. From the start our approach has been

to look at clinical processes and achieve some victories there. One of the things we've gotten into recently is the patient-focused QI plan. We intend to show that it's possible to focus on QI as opposed to QA. If that can be done, then the physicians can be pulled along a lot easier. Through this process, we have engendered the support of five to ten physicians on a multidisciplinary team that's evaluating breast cancer from the moment of initial detection to the time and manner in which the cancer is treated. This team is very large—in fact, it's such a large team we call it the "megawhopper." The team is actually a group of process action teams. We look at every aspect of breast cancer, and the physicians enjoy the process.

Prevost: I recall that the "megawhopper" produced a macrolevel flowchart on the issue of breast disease detection, looking at the patient's course through the institution. Once that was put together, everyone began to see how the various department patient care processes were related and connected. All of a sudden the medical staff saw the importance of systems thinking, and that launched QI for clinicians as well as administrators.

What other kinds of ideas, besides those that deal with systems thinking, get physicians engaged in QI?

Pugh: To get their attention, we look at processes that are long-term irritants for physicians such as medical records or clinical result reporting or admissions—things they battle with on a daily basis. When you show physicians the improvements you've made in those processes, you win a lot of support. We got a lot of support from our physicians when they suddenly realized that they hadn't thought about admissions in three months. They used to think about admissions every day because of the problems they had with the service. As improvements are made, some of these services become invisible.

On our clinical side, we now have physician leadership stepping up and saying they want to make things better. We're doing the same sort of macroflowcharting that John Anderson spoke of for the care provided to a cardiology patient. We have never done this before—looking at the whole issue of how a cardiology patient is sent through the system. We have a lot of physician support for these efforts.

Prevost: Let's touch on one last issue. Attending physicians are not salaried, and there's the problem of time. It's a very practical issue. Tom Wilburn tells us that one has to be very judicious about how we use physicians' time on teams. Are there any other ideas of how to deal with this very practical issue?

Wilburn: We're being very cognizant of the time physicians spend on a team. So, for example, if they need to learn some of the tools, we try to give them intensive, short, just-in-time education. If physicians feel that you're trying to be cognizant of the time that they're spending and helpful in keeping that to a minimum, they're very willing to participate.

Newbold: Good credible data are another catalyst. Physicians enjoy data and if we can provide good credible

data, it won't take a lot of their time to analyze them.

Pugh: There is an incredible difference in the medical staff's reaction when you bring them data that are plotted over time or arranged in a histogram or another simple tool. They'll say, "Oh yeah," and get involved. Before when you brought them data in tabular form or some other traditional way, they'd argue with you, tell you that the data are all wrong. The change has been remarkable.

Newbold: The blame-free environment where people look at work processes and try to figure out the reasons for variation is quite different from what we've had in the past. In the past it was: "Who's this guy here, who's #106 anyway?" The question has changed to "Why do we have this kind of pattern?"

CULTURAL CHANGE

Prevost: We found at the time of our site visits that hospital staff often spoke of a cultural change when describing the organizational transformation to QI. We sensed this change when we spoke to staff and walked around your hospitals. Unfortunately, the use of that expression does not translate readily into an understanding of the concept. The Greek word *metanoia*, meaning beyond the mind, a shift in thinking, or a transcedence to a new way of thinking, might help in understanding this concept. What are the characterist metanoia in this transformation? How do you know when it occurs?

Panzer: One characteristic is a change

in people's automatic, unconscious responses. You can be sure such a change has occurred when an organization's leader walks into a room and staff two or three levels down say, "You're late. Don't you know one of our rules of behavior is that everybody must be on time?" That happened to our chief executive officer the day before yesterday. If this kind of experience occurs pervasively, then I think the kind of change we're talking about is happening.

Pugh: At Parkview, we stopped chartering teams and told managers and everybody else that teams are just another tool, like a run chart or Pareto analysis, that help get the job done. I was stunned the other day when I got a list of teams in the organization—there were 70 teams on that list. I knew of maybe 20 or 25 of those teams. Many are natural work group teams looking at different processes on their own initiative. They haven't gotten together because I said they should, it just happened. This and the physical evidence you see walking through the departments—data plotted over time and posted on the wall, storyboards, and so on—is all an indication of cultural change.

Anderson: Another indication that a cultural change is, in fact, occurring is that all members of the organization, or most, begin to speak through data as opposed to basing what they do on a gut feeling. Staff no longer rely on "factoids" when they have relevant facts on hand.

Newbold: "Factoids?"

Anderson: Factoids. Things that appear to be facts. But they're really a type of opinion that has come to be considered a fact.

Another noticeable indication of cultural change is that staff are employing the scientific method, whether you're talking about using the FOCUS-PDCA approach or some other approach that is consistent with CQI. You know that the CQI philosophy is infiltrating the organization when staff focus on PDCA, look at processes, and stop blaming people. At this point, you can be fairly assured that you're moving in a positive manner toward that TQM culture.

Wilburn: We've set up a team to specifically address the issue of organizational transformation. The team has concluded that transformation is occurring, for example, when you see managers make decisions that benefit the overall organization, and yet might hurt their personal interest. Another example is employees developing an organizational perspective, as opposed to an individual or departmental orientation, and working with customers and in teams toward total process improvement. Transformation is occurring when employees feel empowered, when they feel encouraged to provide information and be the change agents in actually implementing new ideas and solutions.

Transformation is occurring when decision-making is data driven and when staff are listening to what the customer wants, whether it's an internal customer or an external customer, a physician or patient, a third-party payer or industry. And finally, transformation is occurring when you see a lot of coaching and mentoring going on, when no-fault learning takes place, and when no retribution is reaped on an employee if one of his or her decisions has less than positive results.

Prevost: Are there some QI principles or processes that are most critical in promoting *metanoia*, this cultural change in the individual? From your experience, what are the most important enabling factors?

Anderson: Grasping the concept of the internal customer has been a very significant agent for cultural change. Prior to that, most of us in health care focused on the patient as the only important person that we really had to be concerned about. Once the concept of internal customers became clearly understood, then it became a lot easier to understand the TQM process, to understand that if the internal customer's needs were not considered, you were doomed to have a failed process.

Bingham: I am thinking specifically about Deming's points regarding fear and opportunities for growth. It strikes me that cultural change is about employees being a part of the culture—where they truly have joy in work and when they have the opportunity to grow as people and use their talents. It seems to me that this is the "liberation" factor. When the barriers to pride in work are removed in the culture that exists, then I think you're going to start seeing the kind of transformation we're talking about here.

One other characteristic of transformation that hasn't been talked about concerns the idea of innovation. Transformation is not just improvement of existing products and services. You start achieving breakthrough thinking widely throughout the organization when people's creativity is engaged. When this happens, then I think you have cultural transformation or a *metanoia*. I've seen a lot of people focus on improving processes rather than employing innovation. When breakthrough thinking is pervasive throughout the organization, then we will have transformed our cultures.

Prevost: The term *empowerment* has been used and, yet, I personally feel that I don't have a grasp on what it means. Should I see empowerment as synonymous with *metanoia*? Is empowerment part of cultural change?

Newbold: Empowerment is a complex subject. But, to begin, I would say that empowerment is a fundamental belief and trust in the worth and dignity of people. Everybody would agree with that, but whether they demonstrate that belief in their behaviors is really more the issue. Our nurses have been into empowerment for some time now, and they developed a whole system of beliefs, a credo, long before we got into TQM. This belief system addresses behaviors, ways of thinking and treating people, and the concepts of self-worth and self-esteem.

If someone had described such a belief system to me ten years ago, I would have said that it had absolutely no place in an organization. Staff should leave their troubles at the door. They get paid well, have great benefits, and good working conditions. Management is not here to change people's lives. Yet, now it is difficult to introduce TQM when people have grown up feeling powerless in their work and professional careers, when they didn't have any degree of control over what they did. This is particularly relevent when dealing with nurses. Their training was often very task oriented, they were dominated by medical staff, their training was often very domineering by their faculty. When people suffer from low self-esteem, and the chief executive officer says, "All the old rules are off now. We want you to serve on teams and contribute. You're the expert. This is the work that you know best. Here's the sword, go sic 'em," staff respond, "Now, wait a minute. I'm not sure if I want to do that, if I'm capable of doing that." There are a lot of issues having to do with self-esteem, how they fit into the work group, their role as the caregiver, and so on involved in this.

We found that it's taken a lot of time and effort and training on empowerment. It's made a really big difference, but empowerment is the most elusive, softest stuff I've ever run up against. It just drives our board members and physicians crazy to listen to all the issues that fall out of this empowerment philosophy. And yet, it's probably the strongest thing that's holding the nurses together in our hospital right now. I'm convinced that empowerment has really made a big difference in how we've done as an organization in the past three to five years. We've had lower turnover and vacancy rates and begun shared governance and self-managed work groups—all of which has sprung out of empowerment. It's really amazing.

Pugh: I agree with Phil that empowerment is a "soft term." There are no very good operational definitions of empowerment. In fact, there are even some negative connotations. We joke when we talk about "empowering" people in our organization, when we really mean somebody got dumped on. Empowerment and delegation are not the same thing.

Empowerment is not an egalitarian process. In some ways empowerment leads people to look for false paths because they believe that empowerment means everyone is equal. That isn't how it works. I see quality as being very much a leader-driven approach at all levels of the organization, not just the senior leaders, but department leaders, shift leaders, team leaders, and so on.

The reason TQM must be leader driven goes back to the underlying theory of variation, which says it is management's job to change the system. They are the ones who are empowered to change the system. They have the resources, the tools, and the power to make the changes. The people who work in the system need to be empowered to take care of those special causes that occur in their day-to-day job. Management wants staff to be able to fix those problems as they occur as well as participate in efforts to improve the overall system. The things you teach about quality at the line level may be different than what you teach managers. Maintaining that empowerment means everybody is equal can lead people down a false path.

Prevost: Do the rest of you agree with Michael's comment?

Anderson: Not quite. From the managerial side, we're looking at the macroview of how all this fits together. I really think that the employees close to the process have a much better idea of the process than we do. However, those employees don't have a clue how those processes fit into the whole organization. That's our job as managers—to apply the information and improvements we gain from staff toward improving the whole organization. That's really where the difference is. It must be recognized that empowerment allows staff to feel they can make a significant difference, but that management has control over that process. Our job is to be mentors to staff, and as I said, to synthesize their improvement efforts in the multiple processes of the hospital.

Prevost: How do you, as the leaders, keep your fingers on the pulse of the organization's progress with the cultural change you wish to occur? Can you measure this progress?

Wilburn: One of the things that you look for, at least in the early stage, is whether management's behavior is congruent with TQM philosophy and principles. If it isn't, you can throw empowerment and all the other good things out the window. The impetus for setting the organization's tone is the same as the implementation of TQM—it's driven from the top down. And consistent behavior on the part of the management group is one of the most significant things that has to be watched. If it isn't occurring, progress isn't occurring.

Recently a senior vice-president criticized a spontaneous project that a team wanted to take a shot at. He came back two weeks later and apologized. He said to the team, "You know,

I made that criticism because I had tried to solve that problem myself and couldn't, and I figured if I couldn't do it, you couldn't do it. I didn't realize until after I'd made the criticism that I'd taken a very short-sighted approach to it." If behavior such as his is occurring in an organization, I think you're getting change.

Bingham: More and more I ask employees "How does what you do on a daily basis line up with our vision?" For example, three members of a team went to a Hastings Institute conference on biomedical ethics to help them with a project dealing with decisions near the end of life. When I asked how attending this conference related to our vision, they were able to articulate how it lined up. You can ask that same question about a computer system, a clinical practice model, a delivery system in nursing— almost anything. The extent to which staff can relate what they're doing to our hospital vision tells me whether we're achieving a conversion.

Newbold: Tom Wilburn's comments on role modeling, particularly the behaviors of leadership or management, are most important. Ghandi once said "you must be what you want to see happen." The fact that we, as managers, can behave one way in one setting and a different way in another setting is the biggest tip-off that we don't exactly practice what we preach. We send out so many tip-offs and signals every day. We have to watch ourselves, ask for feedback on our behavior.

Panzer: An organization should measure two things to determine cultural transformation. First, what does management do during their senior-level meetings? What do they talk about? Do they talk about customers, about quality, or do they first talk about finances. Second, what evidence is there that individual and team behaviors are spontaneous and not forced from above? If you had a feel for these two ends of the spectrum, you'd probably have a pretty good idea of what was happening in the organization.

INSTITUTIONALIZING QI

Prevost: If the transformation to a QI culture in a hospital is a top-driven transition and the chief executive officer is the usual catalyst, what steps will ensure the continuation of the process if leadership changes? I'm going to ask John Anderson to begin the discussion on this issue because he's participated in such a change at Wright-Patterson.

Anderson: In the military reassignment occurs fairly frequently, probably every two to three years. Commanders move around for several reasons—someone may retire, somebody goes into something else, or somebody is recognized. This happened at Wright-Patterson. The person who really was the initial catalyst for TQM was Colonel Roadman. He got Wright-Patterson started on TQM and then he was reassigned.

When I found out from headquarters that they were going to assign me to be the new commander at Wright-Patterson, I was very pleased and flattered because it's one of the flagship operations in the Air Force. Shortly after, I received a telephone call from one of the senior executives at the

medical center who said, "Sir, we're looking forward to your arrival, and we know that you're going to enjoy Wright-Patterson. And, by the way, we hope that you don't want to change our management philosophy. We believe that TQM is the way that we should do things and we hope that you don't want to come in and change that."

What option did I have other than to say, "Of course not." I understand leadership very clearly. If you're going to lead someone, you've got to have someone behind you. If they're all out ahead of you, you won't be leading very long. So, when I hung up, I began to look more closely at TQM. That was the motivation for me to get very deeply involved in TQM.

Newbold: If any of us chief executive officers went to a new organization, we'd naturally want to put our own stamp on it. We'd want to have our own spin on things. It's pretty hard to be against quality. You're on the side of the angels when you talk about quality. It has more to do with someone doing things a little bit differently than your predecessor.

Look at Rod Wolford who took over NKC or Alliant in Louisville, Kentucky. He continued the QI effort, and he just put his own stamp on it. I'm doing a board retreat for an organization that is going through an administrator change. They're thinking about adopting TQM first and then recruiting an administrator after that, which is an interesting approach.

All of us would like to have our own way of doing things. When I came to Memorial, the organization was heavily into guest relations. I probably twisted the jargon a little bit and used a little different approach. I think that's institutionalization—feeling a sense of ownership and having some influence on the way TQM is rolled out in the hospital.

Wilburn: John Anderson's comment reminds me of a quote by Disraeli. He said, "Of course I must follow the people, am I not their leader?" I'm probably the oldest chief executive officer here, so I'm thinking about succession planning. That's probably a good thing for every leader to do; it probably ought to begin the day you start the job. We're drawing on opportunities inside our organzation, developing a future administrator from within our senior management rather than looking outside the organization for candidates. An internal candidate that has already adopted the TQM philosophy, is participating in the movement, and will continue it.

Anderson: The governing board has to be involved in TQM training and education very early on. Doing that will assure the continuity that we're looking for.

Another approach that I've heard of, and I think we've even experienced to some degree, is to have a TQM champion within the organization. Then, even if the chief executive officer leaves, you have a significant person in the organization, someone who is strong and influential, who will encourage and stimulate staff and leadership to continue on the TQM path. This person can help you in the interim while you're making a transi-

tion in leadership.

Pugh: The individuals on the governing body who have, through their own industries, experience with QI are big stimulaters and also provide some insurance of maintaining the hospital's transformation. If I should leave, get hit by a truck, or whatever, the board would look for a replacement that shares the same sort of values and approach to quality as I have. The board ultimately may be the strongest link to the ongoing movement because they're the ones that are going to make the decision about my successor.

EXTERNAL ENVIRONMENT

Prevost: What are the external environmental factors, whether they be social, legal, political, or economic, that impact both your own hospital's transition to QI and the overall transition within the health care industry, either in a positive or a negative way?

Newbold: One factor is the payment system, which only pays for fixing things after they are broken. There's very little investment in prevention. This is the acute care model that we work in. These difficulties with the payment system drive a lot of the behaviors that engage hospitals.

Bingham: I'd like to comment on the RBRVS [Resource-Based Relative Value Scale]. Is it budget neutral or is it in fact a cost cutting system that they're putting in place? And what will this do to our medical staff in terms of their attitudes toward treating Medicare patients? There is also the whole identity crisis that physicians will be going through in the next few years. What is their role? Are they gatekeepers or partners with hospitals? Are they independent? Must they be entrepreneurs? The payment system is really going to bring these issues into sharp focus.

Pugh: One of the things I see as a major problem is the faddishness of health care management. We shift from one management model to the next, and in the interim language and meaning become confused. At lunch Phil Newbold commented that in Japan everybody shares the same language for QI. People have the same operational definitions and so they can communicate more easily. We don't have that here in the United States. There's a lot of confusion. To give you an example of the confusion, this Joint Commission pencil I am holding reads "Celebrating 40 Years of Quality Improvement." My operational definition of QI is somewhat more specific than this slogan.

On the positive side, the fact that the Joint Commission came out a couple of years ago and said, "everybody's going to move toward continuous improvement in quality" provides a great stimulus to the industry. The industry needs this external stimulus.

Anderson: If an organization is involved with a supplier who is also employing TQM principles and/or involved with regulators who are supportive of TQM initiatives, these relationships will help push or propel the organization toward TQM. If the reverse is true, then these suppliers or regulators would hold the organization back.

There are several other positive and negative environmental factors that influence an organization's transition to TQM. On the positive side, we were fortunate at Wright-Patterson to be part of a larger organization, the Air Force Logistics Command, that was already into TQM when we began our roll out. Similarly, success can promote change. For example, the Air Force Logistic Command was the winner of the Presidential Award for 1990, which is the equivalent of the Malcolm Baldrige award for governmental agencies. The Presidential Award success helped propel us to some degree allowing us to effectively benchmark ourselves.

A potential negative environmental factor I want to bring out is a union leadership in your organization who feels threatened by CQI. Although we have not experienced this at Wright-Patterson, I think that this could be of some concern to organizations with very traditional labor-management relationships.

Newbold: We have a union. We share this stuff with them all the time, and it has gone pretty well so far. But I understand how a union leadership could have a negative impact.

Wilburn: As an industry and a nation, we're facing three major issues in health care. One is access, and the others are cost and quality. All those factors are propelling us in the direction of TQM. Obviously, addressing the cost/quality issue is primary. If we solve our systems problems in a better fashion, we will also improve access.

The fact that our customers are becoming more data-driven or information conscious is another propellant toward TQM. All our customers are now looking for data. The industries that we work with and, obviously, the government are all interested in quality information. Currently, data are not very easily come by or very understandable, and we must use outcome information until something better becomes available. Most of the data we see today do not help us in making judgments.

The public is becoming more attentive to quality as well. Business has certainly placed a strong emphasis on total quality in recent years. As you know, companies now advertise winning the Baldrige award. These kinds of methods are bringing quality to the public's attention. In order to respond responsibly, hospitals need data and information that we've never had before. Since hospitals that are moving toward TQM are beginning to derive these data for our own purposes of improving what we do, we'll be in a much better position to answer the public's questions.

I agree that a lot of aspects of the payment system are deterrents. In the short term, I don't know if hospitals will be able to affect this situation. However, in the long term, I believe reimbursement will become more dependent on the quality of the service that the hospital renders. Looking long term, I think the payment system will propel quality initiatives.

Pugh: It comes down to survival. I happen to come from a hospital that is 95% Medicare, Medicaid, HMO, PPO, and medically indigent. We have tremendous economic interest in improving quality. I believe in the Deming Chain Reaction, which says

you will decrease costs when you improve quality. This becomes a tremendous stimulus for organizations to do something.

Patient complaints are another stimulus. People complain about their hospital bills not being right all the time. They're right. Very few patient bills in this country for inpatient stays go through the straight side of a flowchart. If you flowcharted the process, you'd probably find some reworker fixing stuff along the process.

My gut fact, or gut feeling, is that 25%–50% of all costs in our hospitals are due to poor systems that create waste, rework, needless complexity, malpractice medicine, and wrong clinical decisions. This provides a tremendous stimulus for doing something different. Just knocking out a portion of the cost of rework could free up a lot of the dollars for access, prevention, and additional care.

One of the greatest external stimulants is the payment system, and I don't have any expectation that it's going to change in favor of hospitals anytime soon. The destiny of hospitals' fall is in our own hands. It is up to us to make the hospitals better.

Prevost: It sounds like negative economic factors are in fact a stimulus for moving into QI.

Pugh: Absolutely. Bob Panzer made the comment earlier that a hospital in financial trouble should perhaps not take on TQM. I'd turn around and say if a hospital is in financial trouble, it should absolutely take on a TQM initiative.

Anderson: I think they're afraid to take on TQM because of the costs that they can see engendered in the change.

Panzer: What I meant was that a hospital that anticipates financial trouble should take TQM on, but it shouldn't take it on at the same time that staff are being layed off. At Strong, we had to shove TQM to the side for six months or so because of this very situation.

The contradictory and multiple external oversight issues is another factor. We see the Joint Commission as both facilitating and inhibiting, rather than just inhibiting as in the past. In New York State, we have to also answer to the State Department of Health, PROs, HMOs, and countless employer utilization review companies. Everyone with an 800 number from Lord knows where. These agencies are inhibiting in many senses. The central resources that could be deployed for TQM initiatives are squandered on providing for these external requirements. As these external requirements explode, it becomes expensive keeping up with these requirements simply in terms of expanded manpower. It would be nice if we could assign these additional positions to QI instead of what we're actually doing.

Prevost: What advice would you have for the Joint Commission in relationship to your hospital and to the movement in general?

Panzer: I envision a project team composed of all the participants in quality oversight—representatives from the Joint Commission, New York State, HMOs, PROs, and multiple hospitals. All team members would ask "How can we design a more effi-cient process?" I can envision what this improved process might look like. For example, information regarding the quality of care at all hospitals would only be gathered once. Instead of competing for this information, all external agencies would entrust one agency to gather the data or work together to oversee the collection of this information. The same formats and definitions would be used for attaining information so it would not be necessary to have 15 or 20 cookbooks to get the information. Scientific sampling would be used as opposed to everybody developing their own quality indicators.

Prevost: Bringing together all of the external agencies that impact hospitals, including regulators and accreditors, to explore how they might work together to improve quality of patient care sounds like a good idea. What do the rest of you think?

Bingham: I like the idea of bringing all the players together to understand what we can do together to optimize the system as opposed to suboptimizing it like we're doing right now. I think the Joint Commission is the key player to make that happen. I think it can take the leadership role in transforming the current multiple-inspector system. I'd like to see the Joint Commission take the role of a learning organization, sort of like JUSE [Japanese Union of Scientists and Engineers] is in Japan. That organization serves a different role than one of inspector.

Anderson: I think the Joint Commission needs to consider all of its customers. This includes the various facilities it accredits as well as the constituent agencies that comprise its Board of Commissioners.* These agencies are a set of internal customers that are very distinct and very, very critical to American health care.

We've talked a bit about how to get the physicians involved in TQM. The Joint Commission has the American College of Surgeons (ACS) sitting on its Board. Through this relationship with the Joint Commission, the ACS can learn a good deal about the importance of TQM and then take this knowledge back to their physician members. Similarly, the American Hospital Association can learn a good deal from watching and seeing what the Joint Commission is doing in TQM. Because the Joint Commission is comprised of such a large and important constituency, it can can spread the TQM philosophy to them. It can, if you will, proselytize, and thus very effectively help move TQM throughout the entire health care system.

Wilburn: I am encouraged to hear that the Joint Commission is working on a different type of survey, one that is more consistent with TQM. I think that's good progress. It's encouraging because it says the Joint Commission is willing to work with hospitals, that it is "walking the talk."

Bingham: I think there is also a danger of hospitals beginning to practice TQM simply because the Joint Commission says they must. That's what happened to a lot of other QI efforts. The Joint Commission saying we have to do this becomes the reason why we do things. I don't know how to temper this situation, but I would hate to see the TQM movement go that way.

Prevost: I think we're becoming increasingly sensitive to this issue and the other concerns raised in the discussion about our role and, yes, the Joint Commission is changing. We ourselves are involved in a QI implementation and, I think, appreciate the difficulty of the transition. We are also revising our standards and the accreditation process in the context of QI. Clearly, how we proceed with these changes in accreditation must consider the capacity and readiness of health care organizations to manage the journey.

---

* *The Joint Commission's Board of Commissioners is made up of professionals from its member organizations—the American College of Physicians, American College of Surgeons, American Dental Association, American Hospital Association, and American Medical Association. Three public members also sit on the board.*

9 Future Projections

The study of the six hospitals and their course in the development of a quality improvement (QI) environment has resulted in the identification of issues for the future. This includes not only the future steps that are anticipated by these hospitals, but also the potential impact of QI on the health care field in general and the external support mechanisms that may be needed to facilitate the transition to QI by the field.

As noted earlier, the role of the leadership of an organization has proved to be a critical one in the transition to QI. It is assumed that leadership will play an important role in the *maintenance* of an organization's QI environment. This raises two concerns relating to the future.

The Preparation of Leaders

The first is the extent to which there will be leaders available who have the vision and knowledge to stimulate their organizations to pursue and maintain QI. There is presently little in the academic programs that prepares future leaders in health care relating to QI. This is true for administration or nursing leadership preparation, the medical curriculum for physicians, as well as other health professional preparation programs. As a body of knowledge begins to develop through the experience of hospitals and other health care organizations making the transition, this must be woven into academic preparation programs. Also, continuing education opportunities to prepare those already in the field must be further developed to ensure trained leaders to nurture the field in its development.

Surviving Change in Leadership

Only one of the hospitals studied has gone through a change in the chief executive officer since the initiation of QI—Wright-Patterson Medical Center. Important in that transition was the extent to which

241

the commitment to QI had permeated the senior management and department managers in the center. Also important was the commitment of the equivalent of the governing body, the Air Force Logistics Command, of which the hospital is a part.

The departure of the leader "who started it all" is inevitable for all QI organizations. The extent to which QI survives the transition is critical and is dependent on the degree of institutionalization of the process in the organization. Successful and unsuccessful approaches remain to be tested.

This is a significant challenge for the future of QI in all organizations, not just in health care. There are some lessons in industry. As a part of translating QI into health care from manufacturing and service industries, these should be examined. Changes among the leadership in QI health care settings should also be carefully monitored.

Of particular importance in providing for the future is the degree to which the board is committed—"anchored"—in the QI process. When strong involvement of the board has been an essential part of the process, their determination to continue to move forward and to maintain the gains of QI will have an influence on the decision they make regarding a successor to the senior leader. This may prove to be the deciding factor in the survival of the QI effort in a transition.

Commitment on the part of the governing body members, senior staff, department chairmen and directors, and the training level of staff probably all impact on the potential for success in a leadership transition. More needs to be learned, given the pivotal importance of the role of the senior leader that has been identified.

Institutional Focus

While there is variation among the hospitals studied, there does seem to be a tendency for QI organizations to begin to define their role in the community and society differently as they move through the transition. With its emphasis on systems, multiple causation, and the interrelationship of processes, QI focuses on prevention—not the traditional focus of hospitals and many other health care organizations. Such organizations are traditionally focused on fixing things that are broken. In QI, problems are to be prevented through the pursuit of opportunities for improvement before they become problems. Things are to be made better—the organization is then better able to enhance the health of the patient.

As the focus of the organization begins to shift in the transition to

QI, the board and staff begin to think about health care as a system, focusing on the quality of life of the organization's population. This focus leads to concern about other aspects of the community that impact on the health of the population. Thus, the organization begins to become a proactive force in the community for activities that are designed to enhance the health of the people. This shifts the organization's focus from curing *patients* to keeping *people* well.

This shift in focus for health care organizations is bound to have a significant impact on the health care system in general as QI spreads in the field. This may indeed have implications for cost issues in health care, the commitment of the society to prevention, and many other factors that play a role in the health status and, therefore, quality of life of the American people. The logic of the impact of QI on the orientation of the organization, and those providing it leadership, indicates that in the future many, if not all, QI organizations will begin to reflect a broader concern for society.

It has also been suggested that this leads to a new view of competition. With growing concern for the system of resources that impact the health status of a population, organizations will begin to move their focus from direct competition to developing an appropriate contribution by each to the system. Benchmarking and other sharing activities tend to break down the barriers among organizations. Views of other providers in the community begin to change.

As the boundaries of organizations become more permeable, health care will be increasingly viewed as a system—with the patient moving from level to level of care as required by his or her condition. Some organizations will have difficulty identifying appropriate limits in their interest in affairs beyond the immediate control of the institution. In the roundtable discussion some concern is expressed for these limits and the means to recognize them. The development of this broader role by organizations in the health *system* will bear study as QI moves through the health care field.

Of interest is the degree that such changes in organizational focus are due to the transition to QI and what effect other forces in the environment have had. Again, a fertile field for research has sprung up as hospitals begin to move into QI.

Demonstrating the Effect on Quality of Patient Care

During the roundtable discussion, the six hospital leaders expressed concern that medical staff acceptance, particularly in an atmosphere that emphasizes research and the importance of data (for example, an academic health cente) will eventually require that QI demonstrate an effect on the quality of care received by patients—did outcomes for the patient improve in a QI environment?

Controlled studies, benchmarking among institutions involved in QI, and the relationship of QI to medical research will be important in the development of evidence that demonstrates the care received by patients actually improved because of QI efforts. The improvements in processes that support patient care will be significant in demonstrating effectiveness—more rapid turnarounds in laboratory results will increase satisfaction by physicians. It may also actually address the patient's needs through expedition. Research is needed to be able to demonstrate that these improvements in process resulted in improvements in the care received by the patient, and improved outcomes. Adequate support for such inquiry will also be important.

Changes in Organizational Structure

It is not clear from the six hospitals studied whether significant changes in organizational structure must be a part of the transition to QI. Only one of the hospitals reported a change in structure that was designed to facilitate the transition. On the other hand, it is clear that the structure of the organization must be such that QI is not impeded. However, it is unclear precisely what that means.

Research is needed in this area and will be possible as more organizations begin to move toward QI. The development of models for organizational structure that are conducive to a QI transition will be useful in the future.

Computer Support for QI

Several of the hospitals visited either are in the process of developing or have already addressed their needs for increased access to data. The QI system is based on using data to understand and monitor processes. Without good computer systems to support the process, it is compromised in its effectiveness. In several of the organizations, hand generation of data has been a significant problem in efficiently addressing opportunities for improvement.

The future must see sophisticated computer systems that link together all the data sources in the hospital. The integration o financial data systems with those relating to clinical care, patient demographics, purchasing, and so on will be essential. The ability of all who need access to data to be able to gain that access in a timely and efficient fashion will be essential to the full implementation of the QI process.

In addition, commonality of data bases across health care organizations will become increasingly important as a fundamental tool of benchmarking. Not only will hospitals become interested in common data sets for reimbursements and regulatory purposes, but they will also be important to the ability of organizations to develop understanding of quality-of-care issues across settings.

Standardization, accessibility, and comprehensiveness will be needs that the computer system of the future must meet for each organization and the health care system.

Conclusion

As QI continues to develop in the health care field, a number of questions regarding the needs to support the transition, to better understand what works best in organizations, and the impact of the movement on health care in general will continue to develop. Research that monitors these developments and begins to provide answers to the questions will be important to the ability of QI to thrive in the setting.

Epilogue

One hospital profiled in this book, Memorial Hospital and Health System, South Bend, Indiana, was surveyed by the Joint Commission in the summer of 1991, following completion of the case studies on this publication. On the basis of this survey, Memorial received conditional accreditation—a category of accreditation applied to organizations that are not in substantial compliance with Joint Commission standards but are considered capable of timely resolution of identified performance problems. Such organizations are subject to a follow-up survey at six months to reevaluate the areas of concern. Upon resurvey, the majority of organizations demonstrate satisfactory compliance with the standards.

Although Memorial has a substantial track record in successfully applying quality improvement (QI) concepts in health care, the survey results indicated that the hospital did not fully incorporate continued compliance to Joint Commission standards in its QI activities. The hospital agreed to work with the Joint Commission to examine this situation in order to identify lessons learned that may benefit others engaged in the QI transition. The lessons discussed in this Epilogue address the perspectives of both Memorial and the Joint Commission and raise issues of broad applicability, rather than focusing on those issues that were idiosyncratic to the survey of Memorial.

Emphasis on Quality Planning

Quality management includes planning, assessment, improvement, and maintenance of improvement (quality control). Most organizations in this book learned that QI efforts require an effective initial quality planning process. That is, it is important to systematically identify and set priorities for the processes or systems that are to be subject to improvement efforts. This major undertaking may necessitate significant redirection of resources to achieve a successful transition to quality management. Thus, organizations implementing QI may initially concentrate their energies on quality planning at the expense of quality assessment, improvement, and control activities.

Nevertheless, past and current Joint Commission quality assurance (QA) standards (now quality assessment and improvement [QA/QI] standards) continue to place primary emphasis on assessment activities designed to identify remediable problems and opportunities for improvement, and to maintain compliance with performance expectations where performance is determined to be satisfactory. These standards also primarily stress clinical activities and do not yet incorporate a more encompassing perspective on organizationwide QI activities. Therefore, the potential exists for some dysynchrony between standards expectations and organizational priorities regarding the transition to QI.

For a new hospital or service, a natural progression in managing quality would be to focus first on planning and assessment before attending to monitoring and improvement activities. For existing organizations and services this has not been the historical sequence, and past approaches have been influenced by the national consensus reflected in Joint Commission standards that has established a core set of quality assessment and monitoring requirements. During the transition to QI, such organizations may find it unsettling to attempt to maintain quality assessment and monitoring activities that are of acknowledged importance, when previous related quality planning activities have not yet been fully undertaken. Once more in-depth quality planning for the processes addressed in the standards has been undertaken, the assessment and monitoring activities may be modified to better support continuous improvement. A smooth transition from QA to QI involves a broadening of quality planning to incorporate nonclinical activities, explicit concentration on the assessment of processes, more rigorous attention to QI, and more widespread and concerted attention to maintaining the gain—quality control.

The Joint Commission believes that basic quality assessment and monitoring requirements must continue to be met through the QI transition. There remain certain important clinical, managerial, and support processes that require continuing education (for example, drug use, surgical procedures) even though they may not have been subject to the intensity of initial QI planning and assessment activities yet. Thus, what might be desirable in the real world is not always practical in the reality of providing ongoing important patient care services. There are undoubtedly meaningful parallels in certain manufacturing industries that have ongoing quality assessment and monitoring activities, which could not be discontinued during the QI transition so long as the production lines continued to run.

Physician Involvement

The degree and timing of physician involvement in hospital QI initiatives has varied widely. In some, physician leaders have been actively involved from the beginning and, on occasion, have proven to be the most vocal and effective advocates for such initiatives.

Other hospitals have taken a more cautious approach, choosing to defer physician involvement until the QI initiative is more mature. There are several common reasons for this approach. Some hospitals feel the need to demonstrate the effectiveness of new QI activities before seeking to engage physicians, often because of perceived or anticipated medical staff resistance. Concerns also exist as to the potential increased demands upon physician time during the QI transition—a period during which the eventual efficiencies in physician participation have not yet been realized. Finally, some believe that it is simply easier to introduce QI into nonclinical activities, thus increasing the likelihood of early successes.

While the foregoing rationales may have some degree of validity in individual settings, the Joint Commission believes that failure to involve physician leaders at the onset of a QI initiative is a mistake and violates basic QI concepts. QI principles hold that full-fledged success requires the active participation of all—not some—involved parties and that key leadership groups must all be committed from the beginning. Further, as a practical matter, seeking after-the-fact physician buy-in and support, particularly where anxieties about physician resistance exist, is a hazardous undertaking at best.

Although physician resistance to significant change is a reality in some hospitals, such resistance should not simply be presumed. Nor is resistance to change an attribute peculiar to physicians. A greater reality is that QI offers that tangible prospect of relief and positive change from current QA approaches. The Joint Commission believes that this prospect is highly saleable to physicians. The punitive QA philosophy and the frustrations and inefficiencies of QA activities should make almost any alternative more attractive. QI, however, is more than an alternative; it holds great promise for producing win-win situations for all participants. Further, there is already ample evidence that physicians naturally gravitate toward, and will constructively use, credible performance data. Finally, most physicians will recognize the advantages offered by QI in improving the support processes upon which they depend to provide effective and efficient care.

Not involving physicians early QI initiatives also places hospitals a some substantive risk. When this occurs, the emphasis of the Q initiative becomes, by definition, placed on administrative issues conveying an impression and perhaps a reality that clinical issues ar of lesser importance. Indeed, some hospitals may curtail require monitoring and evaluation activities while hoping to convince th Joint Commission of their demonstrated investment in QI activities The Joint Commission believes that ultimately there will be little meaningful distinction between administrative and clinical processes All such processes eventually impact care of the patient. What i needed, however, is continued balanced attention to those factors tha most significantly affect patient outcomes. This requires appropriat emphasis on clinical care, now in a new mode, and necessitate physician involvement.

External Evaluation: Outcome Versus Process

In recent years, questions have increasingly been raised as to whethe external evaluation (for example, by the Joint Commission) should b based solely on evidence of good outcomes regardless of the processe used to achieve these outcomes or whether external evaluation shoul also focus on those processes that are commonly agreed to affec future performance. The Joint Commission believes that both outcome and processes are important but recognizes the desirability of ar appropriate balance in the accreditation process.

The reasons for balanced attention to outcomes and processes ar apparent. While bad outcomes do occur despite the provision o excellent care, it is equally true that good outcomes may be achieve even in the face of substandard care. Good outcomes should not be ; hit-or-miss proposition. Proper attention to relevant processes reduce the element of chance in the outcome equation. In this sense, th emphasis on certain processes in Joint Commission standards i intended to create a preventive medicine environment in hospitals which enhances the likelihood of demonstrable positive results.

The Joint Commission is now engaged in a major effort to reexam ine relevant organizational processes to identify those that should b addressed in its standards. At the same time, it is recognized that thes standards should be sufficiently flexible to offer innovative organizations meaningful latitude in the design of their specific processes. A proper balance of process requirements and outcomes assessment should eventually enable the Joint Commission to make sound judgments on whether an outcome is acceptable as well as whether it is likely to be sustained and/or improved in the future.

Demonstration of Performance

A related question, both for health care organizations themselves and for external evaluators such as the Joint Commission, is how hospitals record and communicate the effectiveness of their QI activities. A hospital involved in QI may not use traditional forms of communication. For instance, storyboards may be used to describe QI activities, or the records of cross-organizational QI teams may be used as a means of tracking QI efforts rather than traditional department meeting minutes. The issue is not simply *how* and *how much* to document, but also *what* appropriately demonstrates evidence of the effective performance of important processes and productive QI activities. The hospital has the obligation to be able to produce evidence of its efforts and achievements. The Joint Commission has the obligation to assure that its surveyors and staff recognize and give weight to the varied forms of documentation.

Terminology

Initially, QI terminology may seem foreign to those accustomed to traditional QA activities, and the terminology indeed varies among different QI approaches. These variations may result in different paradigms that can lead to communication problems between organizations and confusion at the time of the Joint Commission survey.

The Joint Commission recognizes its obligation to ensure that surveyors are familiar with basic QI concepts, approaches, and terminology. Toward this end, Joint Commission surveyors are now receiving ongoing education and training in QI. A related objective is the Joint Commission's expectation that surveyors be flexible and recognize that different approaches do, in fact, meet the intent of the standards (for example, that different process improvement models can be used to meet the standards requirements).

Having said this, it is also a reasonable expectation that each organization be able to describe to the surveyors, in a clear and understandable fashion, the manner in which it is approaching QI and the terminology it employs. This will avoid unproductive diversions from the issues of central interest. What Joint Commission surveyors should be able to focus on is the logical and effective progression of steps used to study and address identified concerns. Such a progression of steps need not follow any specific model.

Use of Data

Likewise, the focus and display of data may be different for QI than for QA. The Joint Commission requires health care organizations to use indicators in QA/QI activities; these indicators have been focused primarily on clinical care, especially outcomes. Organizations involved in QI use a great deal of data in their process improvement efforts, but the data are often formatted differently than indicator data traditionally collected in the monitoring and evaluation process. In addition, the performance measures applied may have a different focus than indicators have had in the past (for example, more on governance, managerial, and support processes). Nevertheless, all would agree with the importance of making process improvement decisions on the basis of accurate measurements and sound data and information. With this understanding, the form that the data takes becomes less important.

Summary

While this epilogue was prompted by the result of Memorial's accreditation survey, the issues discussed herein are already quite evident in many other hospitals engaged in QI initiatives. The Joint Commission's ultimate objective is to improve the performance of health care organizations through it standards and its accreditation process. Both the Joint Commission and a rapidly growing number of health care organizations are engaged in a transition toward new approaches for improving performance.

Through this transition, it is important to recognize that QI is not an end in itself. Rather, its core principles and methods represent an important evolution from traditional QA activities, thus enabling health care organizations to more predictably improve the quality of their work. Joint Commission standards will not require health care organizations to formally adopt QI per se or any specific management style. However, there will be an articulated expectation of continuous improvement in patient care outcomes and in the performance of important organizational processes. To this end, the Joint Commission is selectively incorporating into its standards only those QI concepts that are viewed as essential to the eventual achievement of improved performance. Most would consider QI concepts simply as sound management principles.

As the Joint Commission engages in a major reorganization and revision of its standards, it will become increasingly important to understand the implications of the transition to QI and the relationship of this transition to the standards. It will also be important for the Joint Commission to provide educational assistance to organizations and to provide examples of how organizations have successfully managed the transition.

This book is not meant to describe either the best or the right approaches to QI, nor is there any claim that these organizations have found the optimal way to integrate QI with current standards requirements. It is likely that some health care organizations will experience difficulties in this regard. To the extent that conflicts between standards requirements and the transition to QI exist, or may occur in the future, the Joint Commission believes that the health care field is better served when these issues are addressed openly. We need to learn from each other, and if indeed there are problems with the transition, it is important that they be collectively explored.

Appendix A
An Overview of QI Tools

Quality improvement (QI) tools are one of the more visible signs of QI activities occurring within an organization (for example, flowcharts covering the walls, data shown in histograms or control charts). Although these tools effectively help staff in problem solving and planning activities, they are only instruments for implementing QI concepts (such as an internist using a stethoscope or a surgeon using a scalpel). The true talent lies in the proper manipulation of the tools. This appendix provides an overview of the common tools QI organizations use; space only allows for short descriptions and simplified illustrations. To attain a more thorough understanding of the use and construction of these tools, several resources are available.[1-7]

The Seven Quality Control Tools

Often referred to as the seven "basic" tools, the following tools are primarily used by teams and individuals in problem-solving activities. However, these tools are often useful in planning and visioning as well.

FLOWCHART

"The easiest and best way to understand a process is to draw a picture of it," writes John T. Burr.[8] A flowchart is essentially a pictorial representation of the steps in a process. The idea behind a flowchart is that a process cannot be improved until everyone involved understands and agrees what that process is. After delineating a current process, staff streamline and improve the process by identifying redundancies, inefficiencies, and misunderstandings. Flowcharts can

This appendix was reviewed by Paul E. Plsek, Paul Plsek and Associates, Roswell, Georgia.

also be helpful in identifying points in the process at which data can be gathered to help assess and improve the process.

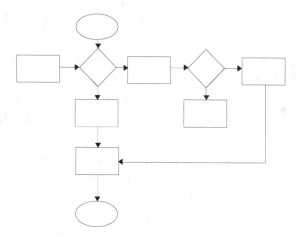

CAUSE-AND-EFFECT DIAGRAMS

This tool helps staff generate and organize theories about the possible causes of a problem or condition ("effect"). This helps staff plan for data collection so they can pinpoint the actual or most frequently occurring causes. The effect or problem is stated on the right side of the chart. Team members then brainstorm on the major influences or causes, which are placed as "branches" stemming from the problem. Causes may be subdivided under broad categories (for example, equipment, staff). These diagrams are often referred to as fishbone diagrams because a well-constructed diagram takes on the shape of a fish.

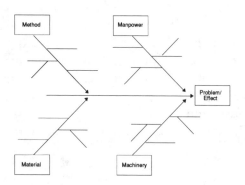

Pareto Charts

Used to identify the "vital few" factors or causes of a problem or situation, the Pareto chart illustrates the frequency of occurrence of various causative events. Named after the 19th century Italian economist Vilfredo Pareto, who observed that the majority of the wealth in an economic system was held by only a few people, the Pareto chart helps teams and individuals decide which factor or cause to address first (that is, their priorities). Pareto charts can be used to identify the most important causes.

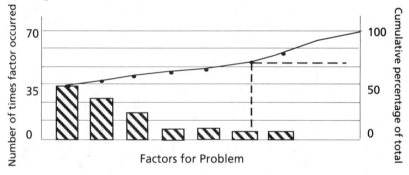

Histograms

A histogram is a graphical display of the variation in a set of repeated measurements from a process (for example, the time it takes to fill a pharmacy order). The height of the bars indicates the frequency with which the measurement falls within certain ranges (for example, X medication orders were filled within 60–70 minutes, Y were filled within 70–80 minutes, and so forth). The overall pattern of the bars—common patterns include bell-shaped, skewed, multiple peaks, and so forth—provide information about the performance of the process that generated the data.

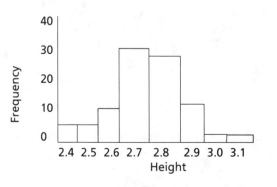

SCATTER DIAGRAM

After plotting data on a scatter diagram, a team can use the tool to explore theories about cause-and-effect relationships between variables. The direction or "tightness" of the dot clusters provides a clue to the strength of the relationship between two variables. However, the scatter diagram cannot, by itself, prove that one variable in the process is causing the change in the other variable. The team must go on to investigate the relationship and acquire deeper knowledge about the process.

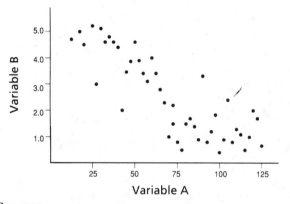

RUN CHART

Used to identify problems and trends within a process, run charts can aid in the study of variation within a process or assess the effect of actions taken to improve a process.

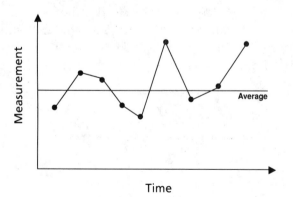

CONTROL CHART

The upper and lower limits are determined by allowing the process to run untouched and then using the data, along with standard statistical models (for example, the normal distribution), to estimate the standard deviation that would result if only common causes were present. By convention, the control limits are then set at 3 standard deviations above and below the average.

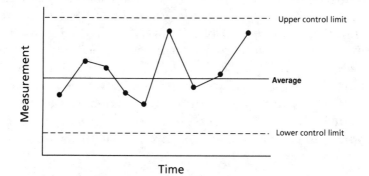

The Seven Management Tools

The following tools are often used in planning and strategic decision making. While many of these tools are also useful in problem solving, managers will find them useful in prioritizing tasks and reaching consensus.

AFFINITY DIAGRAM

This tool is useful when a group needs to sort out the major themes from a large number of ideas, opinions, or issues. When brainstorming, ideas are written on small cards or adhesive notes and then grouped with like ideas and sorted by category.

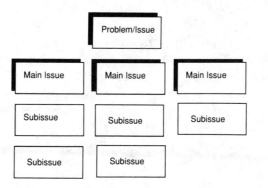

INTERRELATIONSHIP DIAGRAPH

As its name suggests, the interrelationship diagraph helps a team or individual determine the primary cause-and-effect links among issues, tasks, or problems. While the end result looks extremely complicated, this tool is relatively easy to construct and consists of two stages. First, a group brainstorms and puts up all the ideas on small cards or adhesive notes. Then, the group goes back through each card and determines whether it caused or influenced other cards. Once all of the cards have been analyzed, the group identifies those cards with many arrows pointing into, or out from, them. A double box is drawn around all such cards. Cards with many arrows pointing *into* them are key *effects*, which might be measured, while cards with many arrows pointing *out* of them are key *causes*, or "drivers," which should be addressed or monitored. Of course, the relationships shown on the diagram merely represent the opinions of the team members; data may need to be collected to confirm key relationships before major action is taken.

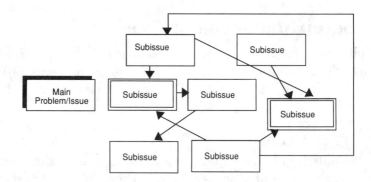

TREE DIAGRAM

Teams use this diagram to show increasing levels of detail under a broad topic. For example, a team might wish to map out the specific tasks that need to be done in order to accomplish some broad objective. First, the team breaks down the primary objective or problem into more workable goals. This can be done using the affinity diagram or by brainstorming. Each subgoal then becomes a major tree heading. For each subgoal, the team asks "what needs to happen or be addressed to resolve or achieve this problem or goal?" The team keeps asking this question until the broad or general tasks become more specific and workable.

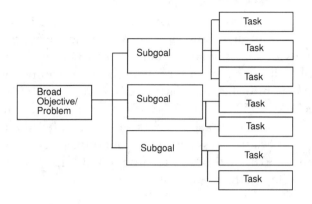

MATRIX DIAGRAM

Teams are often faced with a complex, interrelated, and difficult-to-understand array of tasks, goals, criteria, structures, and so forth. Matrix diagrams can help a team sort out and think through such situations. Items are placed as row and column headings in a grid. The grid can then be used to hold symbols summarizing the team's understanding of the interrelationship between the items. In the example below, a T-shaped matrix is used to show the relationships between a list of tasks, criteria for success, and the various departments in the organization. A square indicates a very strong relationship, a single circle indicates a moderate relationship, a triangle indicates a weak relationship, and a blank space indicates no relationship. For example, the first task is moderately related to the third success criteria, weakly related to the second criteria, and not at all related to the first criteria. Furthermore, this first task requires the strong involvement of department 1, weak involvement from department 2, and no involvement from department 3.

Criteria			▲				
Criteria	▲	■	•	■			
Criteria	•	■		▲			
	Task	Task	Task	Task	Task	Task	Task
Dept 1	■	▲	■	▲		▲	
Dept 2	▲	•	▲		▲		
Dept 3							•

PRIORITIZATION MATRICES

A prioritization matrix is a special type of matrix used for developing consensus on priorities among options. A numerical technique replaces the symbols in the standards matrix (described in the preceding paragraph), allowing more discrimination among competing options. Constructing a prioritization matrix employs a variation of the nominal group technique (NGT), which is a selection process commonly used by teams. In NGT, a team selects criteria (for example, speed, location, timeliness) to evaluate tasks, issues, or options against. Prioritization matrices expand upon the NGT technique and help teams analyze the most desirable or effective options.

Option/ Criteria	Criteria (1.50)	Criteria (1.00)	Criteria (.50)	Total
Option 1	4(1.50) = 6	2 (1.00) = 2	3(.50) = 1.5	9.5
Option 2	2(1.50) = 3	4 (1.00) = 4	1(.50) = .5	7.5
Option 3	3(1.50) = 4.5	1 (1.00) = 1	2(.50) = 1	6.5
Option 4	1(1.50) = 1.5	3(1.00) = 3.0	4(.50) = 2	6.5

PROCESS DECISION PROGRAM CHART (PDPC)

The PDPC is used during planning stages to determine potential contingencies that might occur in an implementation plan as well as appropriate countermeasures. Similar to constructing a tree diagram, staff stop after they list the first or second level of steps they need to perform to achieve a specific objective. They then ask "what unexpected path could this step take?" After all potential obstructions are identified for each task, possible countermeasures are identified and rated. The PDPC allows staff to ask up front "what could go wrong?" and choose the path of least resistance. A numerically coded outline format can also be used rather than the graphic diagram, which is illustrated below.

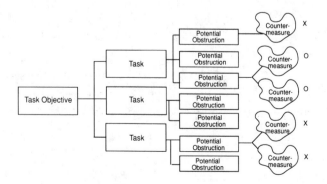

ACTIVITY NETWORK DIAGRAM

This is a tool for planning and monitoring a sequence of tasks over time, showing both the activities required to complete a complex job and the estimates of the amount of time that will be needed for each activity. By adding up the time estimates, the team can estimate the total time required, identify critical paths, and coordinate the timing of parallel paths. The time estimates can also be used to monitor progress during the execution of the tasks

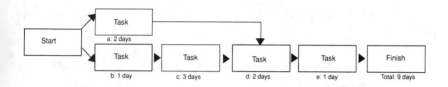

Meeting Management Skills

Many QI organizations have found the following tactics useful in conducting more effective meetings[9]:

- An agenda is set for each meeting with a clear objective defined.

- Participants are assigned roles of leader, recorder, timekeeper, and facilitator.

- Time limits are set for each agenda item (for example, 12 minutes). The timekeeper notifies the leader if the time is up for a particular topic. Participants may decide to "borrow" time from another agenda item.

- Rules of conduct are agreed upon. The facilitator ensures these rules are followed at each meeting. Rules might include

  — arriving on time for meetings;

  — conducting side conversations is not allowed;

  — reaching consensus on decisions; and

  — sticking to the subject (for example, no one is allowed to speak just to hear himself or herself talk).

- Each meeting is evaluated by all participants. During the last five to ten minutes, participants discuss the positive and negative aspects of the meeting, including accomplishments and adherence to the rules of conduct.

- A meeting format is sometimes used to help guide the meeting and help the recorder keep minutes. The format that Wright-Patterson Medical Center uses is provided below.

Meeting Worksheet

Date	Team
Time	

Time (minutes)	Clarify objective		

	Review roles	Leader	Recorder
	Review agenda	Facilitator	Timekeeper

	Work through agenda items
	1.
	2.
	3.
	4.
	5.
	6.
	7.

	Review the meeting record
	Plan the next agenda
	Evaluate the meeting

Agenda outcome/action taken/notes
1.
2.
3.
4.
5.
6.
7.

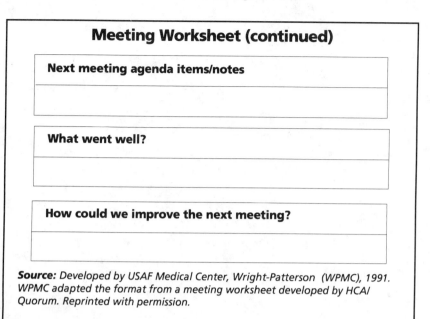

Meeting Worksheet (continued)

Next meeting agenda items/notes

What went well?

How could we improve the next meeting?

Source: Developed by USAF Medical Center, Wright-Patterson (WPMC), 1991. WPMC adapted the format from a meeting worksheet developed by HCA/ Quorum. Reprinted with permission.

References

1. Plsek PE, Onnias A, Early JF: *Quality Improvement Tools.* Wilton, CT: Juran Institute, 1988.

2. GOAL/QPC: *The Memory Jogger: A Pocket Guide of Tools for Continuous Improvement.* Methuen, MA, 1988.

3. Brassard M: *Memory Jogger Plus, Featuring the Seven Management and Planning Tools.* Methuen MA: GOAL/QPC, 1989.

4. Ishikawa K: *Guide to Quality Control.* Tokyo: Asian Productivity Organization, 1976.

5. Western Electric: *Statistical Quality Control Handbook,* 2nd edition, Indianapolis, IN, 1958.

6. Wadsworth HM, Stephens KS, Godfrey AB: *Modern Methods for Quality Control and Improvement.* New York: John Wiley & Sons, 1986.

7. The tools of quality: A seven-part series. *Quality Progress,* Jun-Dec, 1990.

8. Burr JT: The tools of quality, Part 1. Going with the flow(chart). *Quality Progress* 23(6): 64, June 1990.

9. Scholtes P: *The Team Handbook.* Madison, WI: Joiner Associates, Inc, 1989.

Appendix B
Screening Questionnaire

As explained at more length on page 4, an initial list of 60 hospitals implementing quality improvement (QI) was narrowed down to 20 after a review by experts. Nineteen of the 20 hospitals agreed to participate in the next step of the selection process—a structured telephone interview. The following questionnaire was used during this interview to obtain information regarding the extent of each hospital's QI activities. The questionnaire was formulated based on knowledge gained from organizational research and literature reviews on QI. Each interview lasted approximately one hour and involved the chief executive officer of each hospital and/or other key staff. After all the interviews were conducted, the 19 hospitals were evaluated based on criteria provided on pages 5–6, and the 6 hospitals profiled in this publication were selected.

A. Demographics

Number of beds: _____   Average census: _____
Type of hospital: community   teaching   specialty   military
Scope of services: _____
Ownership: not for profit   investor owned   government

B. Organization Involvement in QI

1. How long has the organization been involved in QI?
2. How was involvement in QI initiated?
   Prompts:

   • Was the organization experiencing specific problems (for example, turnover, payer concerns, mortality rates)? Was it a philosophical decision?

   • Was it a top-down effort? What individual/department served as the catalyst for change?

   • How did the organization initially become involved (for example, attended a seminar, required by parent organization)?

- Was a consultant used to initiate efforts?

3. At what stage is the organization in implementation?
4. What percentage of the organization's departments are using QI methods?

C. Leadership Involvement

1. Describe the individuals included in the organization's top leadership. Who has overall responsibility for QI (for example, chief executive officer, chief operating officer, vice-president for quality)?
2. How is the organization's leadership personally involved in QI?
2a. How is management involved?
   Prompts:

   - Is senior management involved in a QI steering committee or council?
   - What percentage of time does the chief executive officer and other senior management spend on QI?
   - Does senior management engage in its own process improvement activities?
   - Does management specifically identify resources or time for QI activities?

2b. How is the governing body involved?
   Prompts:

   - Does the board provide resources or direction for QI efforts?
   - Are QI issues reviewed at board meetings?
   - Does the board receive QI training?
   - Is there other involvement of the governing body (for example, participation in staff training, involvement in its own QI activity, attendance at team meetings, participation on the Steering Committee)?

2c. How is the medical staff involved?
   Prompts:

   - Are the elected/appointed leaders of the medical staff represented on the Steering Committee?
   - Are QI issues reviewed at medical staff executive committee meetings?
   - Is there a special role in QI for the vice-president of medical affairs (employed position if applicable)?

2d. How are other clinical leaders involved (for example, nursing, clinical department heads)?
Prompts:

- Are these leaders represented on the Steering Committee?

D. Customer/Supplier Relationships

1. How are judgments of internal (employees, physicians) and external (patients, families, payers) customers sought concerning the quality of the organization's activities?
Prompts:

- How is information gathered (for example, surveys, focus groups)?
- Are resources specifically allocated for this activity?
- How is this information used? Is it used to establish organizational priorities for QI activities?

2. Are QI relationships established with suppliers?
Prompts:

- Are QI issues included in contractual agreements?
- Are employees of contract services included in the organization's QI activities?
- Do supplier representatives serve on QI teams?

E. Strategic Quality Planning

1. Does the organization's mission statement (describing the business of the business) reflect commitment to QI?
2. Is there a written vision statement (that is, description of a desire future state)? Does it demonstrate commitment to QI?
3. Are objectives designed to reach the vision reflected in annual and long-term plans?
4. How are such plans developed?
5. Is the organization involved in benchmarking (looking at best practices within and outside health care to identify opportunities for improvement)?
6. How is achievement of these plans monitored?
7. Do these plans identify the allocation of resources for QI?
8. Do staff understand the connection between their work and the vision statement/plans? How does the organization assess staff's level of understanding?

. QI Process

1. What is the organization's approach to assessing and improving important processes? How is the Shewhart cycle applied? Are the

outputs of key processes monitored on an ongoing basis?
2. What QI tools are used? How are data displayed and analyzed over time?
3. Are teams used to address process improvement efforts? Are trained facilitators used?
4. What is the relationship between QA and QI?
Prompts:

- Are QA and QI separate functions?
- Has there been an attempt to integrate QA and QI?
- Does QA support or serve as part of QI activities?

G. Quality Results
1. What process improvement activities are currently being conducted? Is the focus mainly on administrative or patient care processes or a combination of both?
2. When variation from expected outcome is found, what action is taken (for example, evaluate system design, assess individual performance)?
Prompts:
If control charts are mentioned,

- how are upper and lower control limits established?
- have there been any breakthroughs in reducing the mean (identifying common causes)?
- how are special causes handled?

3. What successes have been achieved to date?
4. What QI activities have interested physicians?

H. Information Management
1. What types of information are included in the organization's information systems (for example, financial, clinical, patient satisfaction, process measurement)?
Prompts:

- Is this information collected on an ongoing basis?
- Are these systems integrated?
- Are these systems automated?

2. How much staff access is there to this information? Are there limitations on access?
3. Do information systems support team activities?
4. Are data on cost/savings of QI activities collected?

I. Human Resources

1. What types of QI training are provided to staff?
   Prompts:

   - What percentage of staff have received initial training?
   - Are advanced courses provided?
   - Is ongoing training planned?
   - Is there special training for teams/different levels of staff?
   - Are physicians trained in QI methods an tools?
   - Where did staff training begin (for example, with senior management, middle management)?
   - Does senior management actively participate in staff training?

2. Is the organization reexamining personnel policies in terms of QI?

3. How is QI involvement recognized and/or rewarded within the organization?

Appendix C
A Bibliography of QI Resources

Berwick D: Continuous improvement as an ideal in health care. *N Engl J Med* 320: 53-56, 1989.

Berwick D, Godfrey AB, Roessner J: *Curing Health Care.* San Francisco: Jossey-Bass, 1990.

Camp R: *Benchmarking.* Milwaukee: American Society for Quality Control Quality Press, 1989.

Crosby P: *Quality Is Free.* New York: McGraw-Hill, 1979.

Deming WE: *Out of the Crisis.* Cambridge, MA: Massachusetts Institute of Technology Press, 1986.

Feigenbaum AV: *Total Quality Control.* New York: McGraw-Hill, 1983.

Garvin DA: *Managing Quality: The Strategic and Competitive Edge.* New York: The Free Press, 1988.

Gitlow H, Gitlow S: *The Deming Guide to Quality and Competitive Position.* Englewood Cliffs, NJ: Prentice-Hall, 1987.

GOAL/QPC: *Better Designs in Half the Time: Implementing Quality Function Deployment.* Methuen, MA, 1989.

IBM: *Process Control, Capability, and Improvement.* Thornwood, NY: IBM Quality Improvement Education Center, 1986.

Imai M: *Kaizen: The Key to Japan's Competitive Success.* New York: Random House, 1986.

Ishikawa K: *What is Total Quality Control?* Englewood Cliffs, NJ: Prentice-Hall, 1985.

James B: *Quality Management for Health Care Delivery.* Chicago:

Hospital Research Educational Trust, American Hospital Publishing, Inc, 1989.

Juran JM: *Quality Control Handbook*. New York: McGraw-Hill, 1988.

Juran JM: *Managerial Breakthrough*. New York: McGraw-Hill, 1964.

Juran JM: *Juran on Planning for Quality*. New York: The Free Press, 1988.

Juran JM: *Juran on Leadership for Quality*. New York: The Free Press, 1989.

King B: *Hoshin Planning. The Developmental Approach*. Methuen, MA: GOAL/QPC, 1989.

Kouzes J, Posner B: *The Leadership Challenge*. San Francisco: Jossey-Bass, 1991.

Laffel G, Blumenthal D: The case for using industrial quality management science in health care organizations. *JAMA*, Nov 24, 1989, pp 2869–2873.

McLaughlin C, Kaluzny A: Total quality management in health: Making it work. *Health Care Manage Rev* Summer 1990, pp 7–13.

Merry M: Total quality management for physicians: Translating the new paradigm. *QRB*, Mar 1990, pp 101–105.

Moran J, Collett C, Cote C: *Daily Management*. Methuen, MA: GOAL/QPC, 1991.

Nadler G, Hibino S: *Breakthrough Thinking*. Rocklin, CA: Prima Publishing & Communications, 1990.

Peters T: *Thriving on Chaos*. New York: Harper & Row, 1987.

Roberts J, Schyve P: From QA to QI: The views and role of the Joint Commission. *The Quality Letter for Health Care Leaders*, May 1990, pp 9–12.

Scholtes, P: *The Team Handbook*. Madison, WI: Joiner Associates, Inc, 1989.

Senge PM: *The Fifth Discipline*. New York: Doubleday/Currency, 1990.

Scherkenbach W: *The Deming Route to Quality and Productivity*. Rockville, MD: Mercury Press, 1986.

Tufte E: *The Visual Display of Quantitative Information*. Cheshire, CT: The Graphics Press, 1983.

Veatch R: CQI Revisited—Clinical Applications. *The Quality Letter for Healthcare Leaders*, May 1990, pp 1–8.

Wadsworth HM, Stephens KS, Godfrey AB: *Modern Methods for Quality Control and Improvement.* New York: John Wiley & Sons, 1986.

Walton M: *The Deming Management Method.* New York: Putnam Publishing Group, 1986.

Walton M: *Deming Management at Work.* New York: GP Putnam's Sons, 1990.

Index

The health care industry is undergoing a dramatic transition to quality improvement management principles— principles successfully used in business for years. While experts like Deming, Juran, and Crosby have written about QI in business, there is a lack of information on the practical application of these principles to health care. *Striving Toward Improvement* fills this void. It provides valuable insight into the health care industry's implementation of QI and offers practical examples to all professionals seeking to provide quality health care.

Striving Toward Improvement presents case studies of six hospitals' search for QI. This book takes you beyond the principles of QI